DR JOAN GOMEZ is Honorary Consulting Psychiatrist to
th Chelsea and Westminster Hospital. She was trained at
      College, London, and Westminster Hospital and
      ed her DPM and MRCPsych in 1973 and 1974
      ctively, and her Fellowship of the Royal College of
      chiatrists in 1982. She is a member of the Society for
      chosomatic Research, and the Medico-Legal Society,
     a Fellow of the Royal Society of Medicine. She has
      engaged in clinical work and research on the interface
      ween psychiatry and physical medicine. Dr Gomez is
      author of three other books published by Sheldon Press:
      ing with Thyroid Problems (1994), *How to Cope with
      limia (1995) and *How to Cope with Anaemia* (1998). Her
      usband was a general practitioner and they have ten children.

Overcoming Common Problems Series

For a full list of titles please contact
Sheldon Press, Marylebone Road, London NW1 4DU

The Assertiveness Workbook
A plan for busy women
JOANNA GUTMANN

Beating the Comfort Trap
DR WINDY DRYDEN AND JACK
GORDON

Birth Over Thirty Five
SHEILA KITZINGER

Body Language
How to read others' thoughts by their
gestures
ALLAN PEASE

Body Language in Relationships
DAVID COHEN

Calm Down
How to cope with frustration and anger
DR PAUL HAUCK

Cancer – A Family Affair
NEVILLE SHONE

The Candida Diet Book
KAREN BRODY

Caring for Your Elderly Parent
JULIA BURTON-JONES

Cider Vinegar
MARGARET HILLS

Comfort for Depression
JANET HORWOOD

Coping Successfully with Hayfever
DR ROBERT YOUNGSON

**Coping Successfully with Joint
Replacement**
DR TOM SMITH

Coping Successfully with Migraine
SUE DYSON

Coping Successfully with Pain
NEVILLE SHONE

Coping Successfully with Panic Attacks
SHIRLEY TRICKETT

Coping Successfully with PMS
KAREN EVENNETT

**Coping Successfully with Prostate
Problems**
ROSY REYNOLDS

**Coping Successfully with Your Hiatus
Hernia**
DR TOM SMITH

**Coping Successfully with Your Irritable
Bowel**
ROSEMARY NICOL

**Coping Successfully with Your Irritable
Bladder**
JENNIFER HUNT

Coping with Anxiety and Depression
SHIRLEY TRICKETT

Coping with Blushing
DR ROBERT EDELMANN

Coping with Breast Cancer
DR EADIE HEYDERMAN

Coping with Bronchitis and Emphysema
DR TOM SMITH

Coping with Candida
SHIRLEY TRICKETT

Coping with Chronic Fatigue
TRUDIE CHALDER

Coping with Coeliac Disease
KAREN BRODY

Coping with Cystitis
CAROLINE CLAYTON

Coping with Depression and Elation
DR PATRICK McKEON

Coping with Eczema
DR ROBERT YOUNGSON

Coping with Endometriosis
JO MEARS

Coping with Fibroids
MARY-CLAIRE MASON

Coping with a Hernia
DR DAVID DELVIN

Coping with Psoriasis
PROFESSOR RONALD MARKS

Coping with Rheumatism and Arthritis
DR ROBERT YOUNGSON

Coping with Stammering
DR TRUDY STEWART AND JACKIE
TURNBULL

Coping with Stomach Ulcers
DR TOM SMITH

Overcoming Common Problems Series

Overcoming Common Problems Series

Overcoming Common Problems

LIVING WITH DIABETES

Dr Joan Gomez

sheldon **PRESS**

First published in Great Britain in 1995 by
Sheldon Press, SPCK, Marylebone Road, London NW1 4DU

Second impression 1998

© Dr Joan Gomez 1995

British Library Cataloguing-in-Publication Data
A catalogue record for this book is available from the British Library
ISBN 0–85969–723–1

Photoset by Deltatype Ltd, Ellesmere Port, Cheshire
Printed in Great Britain by Biddles Ltd, Guildford and King's Lynn

Contents

1

Why Diabetes Matters to You

It's a twentieth-century First World epidemic. There has been an explosion in the number of people developing diabetes, starting in the 1930s and accelerating since the 1960s. Diabetes is on the increase everywhere, but especially in the advanced countries of the West.

One agreeable cause for the enhanced number of diabetics is that, nowadays, those who develop the acute form of the disease in childhood or their twenties don't die young any more. Insulin and modern expertise have seen to that. However, the main reason for the increase is the flood of new cases, mainly among those over 40. In the UK, there are 60,000 freshly diagnosed every year, bringing the total up to around 750,000, and still rising. These people have diabetes and know they have, but there is an equally large number who have diabetes but are unaware of it. The first group knows what to do to stay healthy, but the second set is in deadly danger.

Unrecognized, this disorder can silently undermine your health over many years, then reveal itself when serious damage has been done. For example, diabetes is the commonest cause of blindness in the UK and USA in those under 65. High blood pressure, a stroke or a heart attack can result from diabetic artery disease; so can the need for amputation, and diabetic kidney problems. Nerve damage can bring on pain and weakness in the limbs, and impotence. For women, there may be difficulties in pregnancy and with giving birth, plus dangers for the baby. Finally, a generally lowered immunity leaves the diabetic vulnerable to infections – especially those involving the chest, skin and urinary system.

None of these nasty illnesses are the direct symptoms of diabetes, they are complications. The risk of developing any of them can be all but cancelled if you know that you are diabetic and you've learned the guidelines early on.

Diabetes can affect either sex and all ages from the unborn to the nonagenarian. What is it in our Western lifestyle that favours its development? The relevant factors are:

- living in crowded cities
- fatty, fast foods available cheaply and in abundance, but a relative

1

dearth of high-fibre foods, fresh fruit and vegetables at the same price

- technology so sophisticated that you don't have to budge from your chair to switch TV channels – exercise is no longer a normal part of daily living
- the prolonged use of various medicines that may tip your metabolism towards developing diabetes (for instance steroids, Tagamet and some of the 'water tablets')
- last, but by no means least, is twentieth-century stress: our world is more competitive and less caring than ever before, financial and sexual insecurity haunt many, so much seems to be expected of us, we struggle to achieve more, but time seems to have shrunk – when did you last work in a relaxed, leisurely way?

So, it is no surprise that the incidence of diabetes is increasing.

What exactly is diabetes?

The term 'diabetes' is Greek for 'passing through', because the most characteristic symptoms are unquenchable thirst, leading to constant drinking and the passing of large volumes of urine. The Egyptians described this phenomenon in a papyrus of 1550 BC. Today we talk of diabetes *mellitus*. Mellitus means 'honey-sweet'. It was Indian doctors of the seventh century who first reported a very significant feature of the illness: the urine of a diabetic tastes sweet. We didn't notice this in Europe until hundreds of years later.

In 1679, Dr Thomas Willis remarked that the water of those suffering from 'the pissing evil' was 'wonderfully sweet'. A century later a Liverpudlian doctor, Matthew Dobson, found that his patient's *blood* was sweet, as well as his urine. The patient, one Peter Dickonson, was passing nearly 16 litres (28 pints) of water every day, yet he had been perfectly well until he was 33. Sadly, the only treatment available was purging and blood-letting – disastrous for poor Peter. The sweetness in the blood and water in diabetes is not, of course, due to honey, but to the most important natural sugar, glucose. If there is an excess in the blood, it passes through the kidneys into the urine.

Your life depends on glucose. Your brain cannot function properly without a steady supply. You cannot think or act normally if there is a shortage in the bloodstream, and you die within minutes if the level falls to zero. Your muscles also burn glucose which is their fuel,

2

enabling you to move, breathe and keep that essential pump, your heart, going non-stop. Athletes, therefore, need large supplies of glucose. This is why you see the tennis stars on the Centre Court at Wimbledon taking frequent top-ups of Lucozade, barley water and bananas between sets. The liver can process carbohydrate and protein foods to make glucose and a storage form, glycogen.

For the body and brain to run efficiently, there must be a balance between supply and demand. The rate at which your liver releases the fuel needs to match the rate at which you burn it up. The glucose level in the blood should remain within a reasonable range. Too little is disastrous, but an overload of sugar in the blood is dangerous in a different way. The ill-effects of an excess amount to diabetes. Your kidneys struggle to wash the syrupy stuff out of your system by producing abnormally large quantities of urine. This means that you feel the need to keep on drinking to replace the fluid you are pouring out. Even so, you feel dreadfully dry.

Nature's neat arrangement for keeping the amount of glucose in your blood spot-on is a hormone called insulin. A hormone is a chemical manufactured in a gland – in this case, the pancreas – and it is carried all over the body via the bloodstream. Insulin gets to every part and tissue, enabling it to use glucose effectively. There is a feedback system to monitor how much glucose is being used and the amount available.

Diabetes develops when there is a serious shortage of insulin: glucose mounts up in the blood because it is not being used properly by the tissues. The short-fall of insulin may be a drastic, near-complete failure of production or a gradually developing imbalance between the supply and the need. In the first situation, the sufferers cannot survive for long unless they get some insulin from an outside source. This is insulin-dependent diabetes mellitus (IDDM).

In the second scenario, there may have been particularly heavy calls on the insulin supply over a considerable period, for instance because the person is overweight or has a taste for easy-to-eat, sweet and fatty foods. This is especially risky in someone who is past the resilience of early adulthood and has given up active participation in energetic sport. This slow type is called non-insulin-dependent diabetes mellitus (NIDDM), because, in many cases, what is needed to put matters right is a change of diet and lifestyle. Sometimes this diabetic will also need to take a medicine by mouth that boosts the production of the body's own insulin.

Whichever way the situation arises, if the body cannot cope with such a fundamental matter as the nourishing and fuelling of the tissues, every part is under threat.

Who gets diabetes?

There are an estimated 98 million diabetics in all worldwide, including 12 million Americans. In the UK, about 2 per cent of the general population is diabetic, rising to 9 per cent among pensioners. The statistics are different for the two main types of diabetes.

• *IDDM* One in five diabetics in Britain has this form. Most of them are young, the peak age for the illness coming on being from 11 to 13, with slightly more boys affected than girls. An old term for it is 'juvenile onset diabetes'. There is a variation in the prevalence of IDDM from country to country and race to race, to do with genes, lifestyle, diet, infection and some mystery factors yet to be discovered. It is increasing in Northern Europe and, to a lesser extent, in North America, arising in the winter months especially. Japan has very little IDDM, while Finland has 35 times as much and Scotland's figures, particularly those for Tayside, are nearly as bad. In the UK, those of Asian and Afro-Caribbean origin are the least likely to be affected, while in the USA the black, Hispanic and Asian Americans are less vulnerable than the whites. In Canada, oddly, fewer of the French Canadians have IDDM than the rest of its population and, in the Middle East, far fewer Arabs, proportionately, than Israelis develop it. In the undeveloped countries of Africa, IDDM is rare but lethal – largely due to the unreliability of the supply of insulin.

Malcolm lived in Edinburgh with his parents and elder sister. He was doing well at school until the Christmas when he was coming up to 11. The whole family had had a fluey cold. Then Malcolm's father, a GP, had a coronary. Malcolm was the first to notice, when they were watching television after supper, that his father had slumped lop-sidedly in his chair. He was dead.

Everyone feels thirsty after a shock, but, some weeks later, Malcolm's mother realized that he was still drinking six or seven cans of coke and going in and out of the toilet all day. He looked exhausted and was unusually rude and irritable. It was all put down to the bereavement, at first, but, instead of gradually getting better, like his sister, Malcolm seemed worse and he had lost a lot of weight. The family doctor, his father's partner, tested Malcolm's urine, then his blood. Both were loaded with glucose: Malcolm had IDDM. For a safe start, he had a short stay in hospital and learned the basic facts about diabetes and the technique of injecting himself with insulin. Now he is a lively member of the Young Diabetics branch of the British Diabetic Association. He is looking forward to a BDA cycling holiday next year.

• *NIDDM* Over 90 per cent of the diabetics in Europe and North America have this type of diabetes, and the numbers are increasing steadily. Some of the increase may be good news in the sense that more people are getting tested nowadays who would otherwise remain in harmful ignorance of their diabetes. NIDDM is predominantly a disease found in the highly developed countries, but people from other cultures are particularly vulnerable to it if they are exposed to the Western way of life. Examples in the UK are those of Asian and Afro-Caribbean backgrounds, the groups least affected by IDDM. A quarter of middle-aged Asians in Britain are diabetic. The situation in the States is similar, while in Australia it is the aborigine population that suffers most.

Geographically speaking, Israel is a black spot, and, for the elderly, Holland, Scotland and Finland. Denmark and Australia come off lightly.

The old name for NIDDM was 'maturity onset diabetes' as sufferers are mainly over 30, with 70 per cent over 50. The older you get, the more likely you are to develop NIDDM, especially if you are a woman. Twice as many women of 65 and over are affected as in the 45 to 64 age band. In the younger age groups there are more men with NIDDM, in a ratio of three to two.

Non-insulin-dependent diabetes might sound milder, but it is known as a wolf in sheep's clothing with good reason. The usual symptoms of diabetes – thirst, passing water frequently – may be so slight that you ignore them, but at least half of all those with NIDDM have already developed some of the secondary effects of the illness before they realize that they are diabetic. The problem is that these complications, unchecked, can impair your sight, your sex life or your mobility or harm your child if you are pregnant. Some of the complications, such as heart, blood pressure or kidney disorders, are potentially life-threatening.

Young Malcolm, although he didn't think so at the time, was lucky that his diabetes was so obvious. The difference is like that between an enemy you can see in broad daylight and someone creeping into your house under cover of darkness. Of course, help is at hand once you know.

Georgina was coming up to 55 and afraid of being pushed into early retirement. She loved her administrative job at the college, but they were streamlining the staff and looking for people they could let go. How she wished that she had stayed pencil-slim – the image of youth, energy, efficiency. The chest pain was a disaster. She was trying to run upstairs at the same pace as her 34-year-old, fitness-freak boss when it stopped her in her tracks. The pain was severe, but it passed off in a matter of minutes. That wasn't the point. Georgina felt that she couldn't afford to be seen to be slowing down.

Her doctor told her that it was angina and that he would give her some tablets that would help. Meanwhile, the nurse had asked Georgina for a urine sample, routine in that practice for those over 50. The result of the urine test was confirmed by a blood test: Georgina was diabetic. Now she and her doctor knew the score, there was a great deal they could do to rectify Georgina's glucose metabolism and halt the progress of the heart and artery problem. After a few months of living a healthier lifestyle, and 3 kg (6½ lbs) lighter, Georgina felt better than she had for months. Her increased energy was noticed by everyone.

Georgina's mother had had trouble with her feet for several years before she died suddenly of a heart attack when she was 62. As she had always stoutly refused to have any truck with doctors, no one could say for certain that her leg and coronary artery problems were due to diabetes. Georgina might have had a check-up earlier if she had thought that there was diabetes in the family.

Who should be screened for diabetes?

None of us wants to make a fuss about nothing, but it is appalling to think that there are many, many people with diabetes who are doing nothing about it, because they don't know they've got it. Doctors are becoming more aware of the lurking danger, but, unless you have some definite reason to seek their advice, you may not have a full physical examination until you are past retirement age. It would be too expensive in time and money to screen everyone for diabetes, but you should ask for a check, specifically mentioning diabetes, if:

- there is diabetes in your family
- you are definitely overweight
- you are pregnant and/or you had difficulties in a previous pregnancy or birth
- your baby weighed 4 kg (9 lbs) or more
- you've been plagued by recurrent urinary or genital area infections or itching in that region
- you tend to get boils and other skin infections
- any of the symptoms of diabetes – there can be other explanations for any of them, but they need investigating. They include constant thirst, passing more water, often at night as well as in the day, blurred vision, weakness and fatigue and, in some cases, weight loss.

Screening for diabetes

This means a test on blood taken from a vein in your arm (it doesn't hurt). There are three types of test.

1 *Random blood sugar test* This is taken on the spot with no special preparation.
2 *Fasting blood sugar test* This involves taking nothing apart from water for at least 14 hours, usually overnight (it provides a slightly more accurate result than the first test).
3 *Oral Glucose Tolerance Test (OGTT)* You eat your normal diet for the few days before the test, but arrive for the test without having had anything for breakfast. You sit and rest for half an hour before the test, if possible, then you have a blood test to check the basic level of glucose in your blood. You then have a drink of 50 to 100 g (2 to 4 oz) glucose in water, then you sit, not moving about much, for an hour or two hours. At the end of this time the blood test is repeated, or you may have two tests – at one hour and two hours after having the drink.
The OGTT is the most certain test, and is the one used for mothers-to-be (at about the twenty-fourth week of pregnancy).

7

While finding sugar in your urine may arouse your doctor's suspicions, only by having a blood test can the doctor tell for sure if you are diabetic.

Why all this fuss about diabetes?

After all, it is only one of a huge number of illnesses. But, in fact, diabetes is unique. The essential fault in diabetes prevents the body from carrying out its most fundamental task: nourishing and fuelling of every organ, every system. When this basic metabolic mechanism breaks down, disorders of the heart, arteries, kidneys, brain, sex organs, eyes and other parts of the body can result. The origin of these disorders is often unrecognized. How many deaths from a stroke or heart attack are really deaths from a complication of diabetes? Half the kidney transplants in this country are necessary because of diabetic kidney disease.

Of acute admissions to hospital in Britain, 3 per cent are for urgent diabetic problems, especially among children and the elderly. In the USA, it is 7 per cent. These figures take no account of the *planned* admissions for chronic problems associated with diabetes.

In every developed country, the cost of diabetes bites a sizeable chunk out of the healthcare budget, around 5 per cent – £1.5 billion annually – of NHS funds in Britain. Most of this is eaten up, not by diabetes itself, but its wide-ranging secondary effects. This means that it is politically and financially, as well as personally, advantageous to prevent these secondary effects or to nip them in the bud by the early, accurate detection of diabetes, and by carrying out research to discover and develop better ways of dealing with the disease and its effects.

The St Vincent Declaration

There is no country in the world where there isn't some suffering because of diabetes, yet much of it need not happen. To ensure that it doesn't, everyone needs to pool their knowledge and plan and pull together across national and international boundaries. That's what St Vincent was about.

In October 1989, the top diabetic specialists from every country in Europe, representatives from all their governmental departments of health and, most importantly, ordinary people with diabetes, met at St

Vincent, in Italy and talked non-stop for two days. They were thrashing out ways of saving the 10 million citizens of Europe known to have diabetes and those at risk from long, wearying years of ill-health and an early death because they are still undiagnosed.

The plans they worked out involved taking action on three fronts:

1 prevention
2 early detection of diabetes
3 effective treatment of diabetes and of the secondary problems it can bring on.

The delegates published a declaration of what they hoped would be achieved throughout Europe over a five-year period:

- new awareness of the potential dangers of diabetes among health-care professionals and the general public
- special arrangements for children with diabetes, whose whole lives depend on our getting it right, information and advice for families, teachers and youth workers
- easily available practical training and education about diabetes for everyone concerned, especially diabetics of all ages
- the goal of making people with diabetes as independent and self-confident as possible, with realistic modifications for the very young and the old
- cooperation and communication about research projects, throughout Europe and, ultimately, the world.

Specific targets
These were:

- to cut down the number of new cases of blindness by at least a third, and prevent the earlier stages of damage to eyesight
- a similar reduction in cases of kidney failure
- to halve the number of diabetics needing to have a limb amputated because of gangrene
- to make pregnancy as safe and the outcome as successful for diabetic women as for others
- to eliminate, as far as possible, the other risks of coronary heart disease among diabetics.

9

Every delegate at St Vincent gave a solemn pledge to take strong and decisive action to achieve these aims in their own country or group.

In England, Consultant Diabetologist Dr Peter Kopelman and his team of half a dozen have already made remarkable progress in the London Borough of Newham. For example, before they started, the death rate for newborn babies of diabetic mothers was 17 per 1,000; today it is down to 7. This is despite the fact that Newham is one of the most deprived of London's inner-city boroughs. A series of talks, discussions and workshops is laid on for all new diabetics and established sufferers as necessary. There is seamless cooperation between hospital clinic, the GPs and the midwifery service, each knowing all about what the others are doing. There are also close links with heart, kidney and eye specialists.

An equally successful operation to reduce infant mortality and complications among diabetics is being run in a totally different setting by Dr Allan McCullough and his colleagues, who are based in the heart of rural Durham, where long distances are a major factor.

Research into diabetes

Most of this research has been carried out in the USA and Europe.

The Diabetes Control and Complications Trial (DCCT)

This big, ambitious project was started in America in 1985. It involved 1,441 diabetics in 29 centres. They were aged between 13 and 39 and all had IDDM.

The aim has been to test the best, established treatment against a new, highly intensive method over a period of ten years and to compare the number and severity of the complications developing in each group.

Half the patients have been on the standard regimen, while the other half have had insulin injections three or four times a day or received it by means of a continuous infusion pump. Glucose levels in the blood have been closely monitored.

The results so far show, without doubt, the benefits of the intensive treatment:

- there have been 76 per cent fewer new cases of diabetic eye disorders
- there has been a 54 per cent reduction in the advance of eye problems that were already present

- there has been a 60 per cent reduction in nerve and mental symptoms
- there has been 54 per cent less kidney disease.

The participants are too young to suffer from heart and artery problems, so any effects of the intensive treatment on these complications could not be shown. Oddly enough, there was no difference between the two groups in terms of their emotional state or sense of satisfaction with their lives.

While the beneficial effects of the intensive treatment are beyond question, there are some disadvantages to it. Apart from the additional time and bother involved, there is an increased risk of succumbing to a hypo – a shortage of glucose in the blood (see page 77). This makes the method unsuitable for young children and some of the elderly.

The United Kingdom Prospective Diabetes Study (UKPDS)

The biggest minus point about the DCCT is that it has only been tried on young people with IDDM when most diabetics have NIDDM. As the World Health Organization pointed out: 'its impact is often not fully acknowledged and should attract more attention from healthcare professionals and planners'. That is where the UKPDS comes in.

It started in 1989, and involves more than 5,000 patients, aged between 25 and 65 (the average age is 52), all newly diagnosed with NIDDM. A large proportion already had eye and heart abnormalities. The aims of the study are:

- to assess the effects on the development of the complications of the avoidable risk factors – smoking, being overweight, having high blood pressure, a high blood sugar level and so on
- to compare diet, antidiabetic medicines and insulin treatment
- to work out ways of matching the treatment to the individual.

The results will start coming in from 1995 onwards.

While the intensive treatment of the DCCT is excellent for those with IDDM, it is not certain how valuable it is for NIDDM. One disadvantage of the treatment, as far as NIDDM is concerned, is that it causes over a third of the patients to put on weight, usually about 4.5 kg (10 lbs). This could increase the risks of heart and artery disease in older, overweight people. Nevertheless, it is usually helpful to have the blood glucose level as near normal as possible.

11

Other research

Research is being carried out into tracking down a virus that may trigger diabetes, the role giving babies cows' milk during their first year plays and the possible effects of wheat in some people.

An exciting project centred on the Wellcome Trust for Human Genetics and involving 100 families at hospitals up and down Britain is aiming to find a simple, cheap way of locating two genes newly discovered to be associated with diabetes. This opens up the possibility, in a few years' time, of detecting the risk and preventing the illness before birth.

Professor Gale at St Bartholomew's Hospital in London is trying out one of the B vitamins as a preventative, while the Americans are using very low-level doses of insulin to head off diabetes in people who are considered vulnerable.

Another group is working on the production of an artificial pancreas to provide insulin in as natural a way as possible. In the US, there is a national diabetes education programme with TV slots, talks and pamphlets. In Britain, from 1994, the British Medical Association and the British Diabetic Association have been pulling out the stops to keep us informed, too. With proper management, diabetes is a lion tamed: all that is needed is the knowledge. Read on to acquire it for yourself.

2
What to look out for

You don't need to be a hypochondriac, but you do need to know which symptoms and signs you ought to bother about. A symptom is something you feel, like a headache or dizziness, that is unusual for you. A sign can be detected by someone else and, of course, you are likely to notice it too, such as swollen ankles or a dry, furred tongue. In practice, signs and symptoms are mixed up together and are both things that make you uncomfortable.

You don't welcome them, yet they are Nature's signposts, showing the way to your well-being. Imagine that you are walking along a cliff path. It is not what you want to see, but it may save your life if there is a notice saying, 'DANGER: landslip'. And you must have come across that maddening road sign of an exclamation mark, which warns you of a hazard ahead, but doesn't tell you what it is. Symptoms can be like that.

Sometimes diabetes develops with no indication of its presence for months and months, but, if you are reasonably on the ball about your own body, it will usually give you some hint of the potential problem in plenty of time to take action. With children and those under 30, diabetes is likely to come on quickly, in a matter of days or weeks. In older adults, though, the symptoms may creep up almost imperceptibly, unless you make it a habit to look back over several months to compare how you felt then with how you feel now.

Signposts that point directly to diabetes

Undue thirst This often begins by your wanting a drink in the night, then needing a glass – later a jug – of water by your bed. If you find yourself taking a bottle of, say, mineral water on a shopping trip, or you get into the habit of bringing a couple of bottles of soft drink to work, to top up during the day, this needs looking into.

David was 21, an exciting age anyway, but he had also just started his first job in a City firm. He had always been keen on sport and bounding with energy, but, suddenly, over a few days, it all seemed to drain away. He put it down to anxiety, together with his dry

13

mouth and disturbed nights. He kept waking up, wanting to pass water. This didn't surprise him as he was knocking back an unaccustomed five or six pints of lager in the evenings, as well as tea, coffee, juice – anything that was going – during the day.

After a week, he felt a wreck and he had lost so much weight that his trousers were in danger of falling down.

David was diagnosed as having IDDM and the treatment he was given soon put him back on track.

An older person might find it difficult to make the connection between wanting endless cups of tea from breakfast until bedtime, plus a 'weak bladder', and diabetes starting up or sliding out of control.

Passing large amounts of urine Some men always have to check the whereabouts of the toilet at a restaurant, a concert hall or a shopping precinct. If they are over 50, everyone mutters about prostate problems, but the cause can be diabetes in those under and over 50. Younger women complain if they have to pass water rather frequently, but the middle-aged, often a little overweight, put it down to their age or having had children if they find they have to find a toilet quickly at all times of day and night.

Vinny was five and her Great-grandmother was 85. They both had the same humiliating experience. After years of being 'dry', they started waking up to find a wet bed. It was October, and Vinny had recently started at primary school, so the bedwetting and her unusual crotchetiness were thought to be psychological. Her mother tried giving her nothing to drink after 4.30 pm. This was miserable for Vinny, but it precipitated the vital emergency visit to the surgery when Vinny became dehydrated and obviously ill.

Mabel, Vinny's Great-grandma, had been a fiercely independent old lady, but lately she had visibly aged, both mentally and physically. She was desperately ashamed of her 'lapse' in the night, but, unfortunately, it wasn't a one-off experience.

She had been told some years ago that she was mildly diabetic and that all that was needed was to adjust her diet, which she did. Mabel assumed that what was happening now was part of an inevitable decline into senility. Her daughter could not agree and thought in terms of a 'chill on the bladder'. She insisted that Mabel see the doctor. Mabel's blood glucose level was very high. After taking a small dose of insulin daily, her enuresis stopped and her mind cleared.

Weight loss losing weight without trying is commoner in, but not exclusive to, those under 40. It can be dramatic, with a loss of 3 kg (½ stone) in a matter of days, or it may be 6.5 kg (1 stone) or more over a few months. In the latter case, you may find to your delight, that, say, a suit that was too tight in the spring fits easily in the autumn.

Lorna had this experience. She was 56 and had been a little bit plump until, to her amazement, she lost quite a bit of weight over a year. During this time her appetite was excellent, if anything bigger than previously, and she did not restrict herself. In fact, she developed a particular craving for shortbread and other sugar-laden foods. When she found that she had lost 9 kg (20 lbs) since the same time the previous year, she was alarmed – could this be cancer? In answer to her GP's questions she admitted that she had become 'rather a water cart' and that she was drinking as well as eating more than usual. The doctor said she had diabetes, not cancer.

Indeterminate symptoms

Any of the following mixed bunch of symptoms may arise in one of a variety of situations – some because of diabetes, some as a result of other physical disorders and some for psychological reasons.

Feeling below par You can't put your finger on it, but you don't feel right. You are tired before you have done anything, you feel a general malaise.

Andrew felt so worn out that when he got home from school, he just had his supper and a bath and went to bed. That would have been all right if he had been a schoolboy, but Andrew was the teacher. He was 35. A wife or a flatmate might have reacted to his crawling off to bed early each night, but Andrew had been on his own since his divorce. When he finally thought something might be wrong and sought help, the diagnosis of diabetes, and the knowledge that something could be done, was a turning point.

Blurred vision There are three ways in which difficulties with sight may be due to diabetes. Someone in middle age or older may or may not be aware that they have NIDDM. Blurred vision in this age group is likely to be due to a cataract, which tends to occur earlier in those with diabetes that isn't under strict control. Exceptionally, it can affect a child. Diabetic retinopathy – damage to the lining of the eye – interferes with sight if it is unchecked for many years. The third cause of misty vision is an excess of glucose, not only in the blood, but in the transparent gel inside the eye. This is often the first indication of diabetes of either type, at any age.

> Maggie, 24, had to focus on a VDU much of her working day. She blamed the screen and the layout of the office for her blurred vision. The area of the office she worked in was rearranged and she visited an optician. She found she needed glasses. Although they seemed to help for a while, she soon started having difficulties again. And she felt so thirsty. She had a check-up.

Constipation This is a common complaint, and is often a side-effect of medicines such as painkillers or antidepressants. If constipation develops when you are eating and drinking without restriction, there is a possibility that it is caused by the fluid loss of diabetes. It is worth having a test to see.

Pins and needles in the hands and feet This is the funny sensation you get if you have been sitting on your legs or lying on your arm too long. You can experience this same symptom if you have diabetes. This is not because you have been pressing on the limb, but because the nerves become irritated by the excess glucose.

Infections We all have infections from time to time and, usually, they are promptly dealt with by the immune system. If infections such as bronchitis, cystitis, spots and boils keep coming back or if trivial injuries are slow to heal, it may be because your defences are low. Diabetes can cause this.

> Norah was horrified to find she had that itchy vaginal discharge again. Her doctor had told her it was thrush last time, and that it was caused by *Candida*. The cream he gave her seemed to work at the time, but now it was just as sore and unpleasant as ever and she

couldn't work out why it had come back. It was a relief to know that it was diabetes.

Men with diabetes can get a similar infection with an irritating discharge from the penis. In either sex, the problem only clears up properly when the diabetes is brought under control. Some overweight people can get thrush in the skin folds. This is a strong motivation to lose weight as it will help your diabetes and your skin.

A cough with chest pain at the back or side, especially if you bring up green phlegm, indicates a chest infection. This is more likely if you have diabetes, but, like all these infections, it can occur anyway.

Faintness and dizziness A swimmy sensation, especially on standing up quickly, is often due to low blood pressure. The loss of fluid that occurs in untreated diabetes can cause this. If it happens more than once, have a check-up.

Dryness A dry mouth, sore, dry eyes and the skin losing its normal elasticity if you pinch up a fold could be due to the fluid loss that results from an extra large output of urine.

Sexually related problems A gradual failure to achieve erections is more likely to happen in men who are 50 or over and may be due to diabetes, but there are also other causes to consider. Women may suffer irregular periods as a result of having diabetes or for a variety of other reasons.

Pain and tightness in the chest on exertion – angina – is relatively common in diabetics. It can be the first intimation of diabetes that you notice. The metabolic disturbance can lead to furring up of the arteries, including the coronaries, in those over 40.

Pale patches of skin This curious condition of irregular loss of skin pigment is called vitiligo. It is not a sign of diabetes, but is evidence of a propensity to develop autoimmune reactions. One of these is IDDM, but others are rheumatoid arthritis and thyroid disease. You can have vitiligo without any other problem, but it is a pointer if you develop any of the vaguer symptoms of diabetes.

Reggie was a gym instructor, so wide areas of his skin were on view.

17

Usually vitiligo is more of a worry to women, but, in Reggie's case, the dead-white areas on his tanned skin were an embarrassment; he felt like a map. His aunt used a cover-up make-up for her face, but he would have had to use such a lot that it just wasn't a practical option. His aunt had also developed an underactive thyroid when she was around 55. Reggie was 20 when he went to the doctor to see what could be done about his skin. He was told that there was no treatment, but that the pale skin was perfectly healthy. The doctor thought Reggie looked strained and rather thin. In fact, he had lost weight lately and admitted to feeling washed out. He turned out to have IDDM.

Other times diabetes comes to light Sometimes diabetes comes to light in the course of an insurance medical, a Well Woman examination, or the check-ups more and more firms are arranging for their executives.

Children and diabetes

Youngsters can have diabetes from babyhood or it may develop during their school years. A general failure to do well, to put on weight and sleep contentedly can signal diabetes – or other problems – in babies. Later on, falling behind in height and growth may be a clue. Often diabetes comes on with unmistakable acute symptoms in a child, but there are some like Tim.

Tim was a whiny five-year-old. His mother felt ashamed that he looked so skinny, although she made sure he had plenty of good, nourishing food. At the school clinic, they said that he was 'below the third percentile', which meant that he was undersize for his age. There was no diabetes in the family, so it came as a shock to learn that Tim had it. It meant a tremendous upheaval in the family routine, but it was a relief to his parents to know that there was a reason their son was so miserable and that it was not their fault. Also that there was treatment for it.

If you already know you are diabetic

New symptoms can crop up that you may not connect with your diabetes, yet the answer may lie with your blood glucose level. Any of the symptoms mentioned below may arise and call for a review of your diabetic status, eyes, weight and so on. There are also other problem caused by established diabetes and it is important that you don't ignore them or believe that your diabetes is irrelevant (see below).

Unexplained injuries These often appear on diabetics' feet. You think you have knocked yourself or that your shoe has rubbed without your feeling it, but it is likely to be because of diabetic nerve damage (see page 98).

Numbness This especially affects the hands or feet. This is also due to nerve damage.

Ulcers These are often painless, but can be difficult to clear up. They are a later result of nerve impairment.

Pain in the calves This is sometimes experienced when you walk far. It may be due to smoking, diabetes or there being too much fat in the blood or all three.

Depression and anxiety If this comes over you and there is no cause that you can pinpoint, it can be the effect of diabetes slipping out of control. Very few of us are happy all the time, but a low mood that interferes with your life needs to be dealt with, in whichever way is appropriate.

Difficulty with swallowing and feeling full This can result from the nerves being affected by your diabetes.

Sweating Often in the night or after a meal this, similarly, points to your nerves being affected by your diabetes.

Diarrhoea This usually happens in the night and is also possibly the result of your nerves being affected.

Itchy skin, weakness and shortness of breath These symptoms together may point to a diabetic kidney problem.

Undue drowsiness This may be serious and either due to a lack of glucose (hypoglycaemia) or to a build-up of glucose and ketones (ketoacidosis). The first is an imbalance, there being relatively too much insulin, in an insulin-dependent diabetic, and it comes on rapidly.

The second is the poisonous effect of diabetes running riot, with a shortage of insulin. In this situation, too, the sufferer is likely to have IDDM and will have been feeling ill for several days. Urgent action is needed in either case (see pages 81 and 73.)

When you see your doctor

You will probably be asked the following questions, so think about them so you can answer them accurately.

- How long have you had this symptom?
- Did it come on gradually or suddenly?
- Can you think of anything that set if off?
- Have you ever had it before? If so, what happened?
- Are you on any medication? The following medicines may make the symptoms of diabetes worse or even bring them on for the first time.
  - Prednesol (prednisolone) and other steroids (30 mg is a high dose)
  - Epanutin (phenytoin)
  - Tagamet (cimetidine)
  - Lasix (frusemide) and some other diuretics, in NIDDM only
  - Indocid (indomethacin)
  - Eltroxin (thyroxine)
  - The Pill, unless it is a low-dose type; progestogen-only ones are more likely to cause problems than others
  - Largactil (chlorpromazine) and other phenothiazines
  - Inderal (propranolol) and other beta-blockers
  - Diamox (acetazolamide).

What not to worry about

This long list of signs and symptoms and things that can go wrong may seem intimidating. The fact is that you are unlikely to have more than one or two of them in a lifetime. Symptoms aren't harmful in themselves, but show that your body trying to tell you something. Often it is something trivial, but sometimes it is a clue to an important problem that could be cut short or avoided.

If you have diabetes, it is obviously essential that you should know about it, so that you can make the necessary corrections to your metabolism, following expert advice. You would do as much for your car if it developed a funny noise or wasn't pulling properly. When you are living with diabetes, it is handy that your body sends out friendly reminders if the control is slipping. This is not a source of worry, but, rather, a safety mechanism. You can often avoid your body's needing to remind you by checking your own blood glucose efficiently. This puts you in charge, one step ahead.

One curious long-term effect of diabetes that could worry you, but needn't, is the appearance of reddish-brown marks on your skin. They may be the effects of a long-healed injury or have no apparent cause. They don't indicate anything going wrong, but may take many months to fade.

3
IDDM and NIDDM: the two types of diabetes

There are half a dozen *varieties* of diabetes and two important, but very different *types*. These are Type 1, or insulin-dependent diabetes mellitus, known as IDDM, and Type 2, or non-insulin-dependent diabetes mellitus, known as NIDDM. With either type, the root of the problem is a shortage of insulin. This hormone, or chemical messenger, is manufactured by the beta-cells of the pancreas, a small sliver of glandular tissue near your stomach.

Normally, when you have just had a meal, there is an influx of nutrients, including sugar, into your bloodstream. The beta-cells respond by making some extra insulin, so that the nourishment can be used to best advantage. The insulin sets off several processes:

- in the liver:
  - glucose (sugar) is taken in and some of it turned into glycogen for storage purposes
  - lipids, body fats, are manufactured for storage in other parts of the body
- in the muscles:
  - glucose is taken in to use as fuel
  - protein muscle tissue is made on the spot
- in the fat stores (beneath the skin and in the abdomen):
  - glucose is taken in
  - fat is taken in
  - fat is produced
- in all tissues:
  - glucose is taken in, as required
- in the blood:
  - the glucose level is kept steady.

A lack of insulin *reverses* all this in the following ways.

- The liver goes on making glucose to excess and releases more glucose from its glycogen stores. Instead of making fat, it makes chemicals called ketones, which are poisonous. The sufferer feels ill and may go into a coma or even die, if nothing is done.

22

- The muscles cannot take in glucose so they try to use fat for fuel, and they break down their own protein. Weight is lost rapidly.
- The fat stores cannot take in glucose or fats, so the stores run down by releasing fats into the bloodstream. Arteries may get silted up, leading to atherosclerosis.
- The blood is flooded with glucose, which the muscles and other tissues cannot take in and use. The high level of glucose in the blood is called hyperglycaemia. It is responsible for the feelings of thirst and the increase in the need to pass water.

IDDM

This is an autoimmune disorder. Others in this group include pernicious anaemia, rheumatoid arthritis, thyrotoxicosis, myxoedema, systemic lupus, a form of hepatitis, the skin condition vitiligo and a host of rare conditions (see page 17). There can be a general susceptibility to any of these, based partly on the family genes, but probably an attack by a virus is required to trigger an actual illness.

What goes wrong is that the immune system, which protects your body from invaders such as bacteria, mistakenly identifies some particular body cells as enemies. In the case of IDDM, the targets are the beta-cells of the pancreas, the insulin manufacturers. Over a period of five to ten years, all these cells are killed. You don't notice anything until 90 per cent of them have been knocked out.

Then your metabolism goes haywire. You cannot deal effectively with carbohydrates, fats or proteins. The level of glucose in your blood rockets because, without insulin, your body can't use it. With glucose made unavailable, your body uses its own fat and protein for fuel. This leaves you weak, drained and losing weight. Your body's efforts to deal with the excess glucose produces the classic symptoms of diabetes – lots of urine and consequent thirst to replace the lost fluid. Misty vision is the result of looking through a syrupy medium, which stems from the excess glucose.

If the situation is allowed to worsen, without treatment, the result is the serious illness of ketoacidosis (see page 73), leading on to diabetic coma (a kind of unrousable sleep) and if, still, nothing is done, death. IDDM is not to be trifled with. How it comes on varies, depending on age. Although it is typically a young person's disorder, it can develop at any age.

IDDM in babies and very young children

Robin was a year old. They say that boys are more difficult to rear than girls, but his parents found this little consolation. Robin was increasingly miserable, restless and difficult with his food. He was often snuffly, but it was when he developed a feverish cold that a crisis was reached. The doctor said it was due to a virus, that there was no point in giving him an antibiotic, but to make sure that he had plenty of fluids. Over the next two days, Robin's restlessness changed to listlessness, he developed a faint rash and, far from drinking more, he began vomiting more and more frequently.

He was obviously very ill. Meningitis was suspected and he was given a range of tests, including one for blood sugar, which revealed the problem.

Diabetes is an unusual cause for a baby's poor progress, but the final trigger to severe, obvious symptoms is often a viral illness.

IDDM and school-age children

Adam was an easy child – well-behaved when it mattered and coming along nicely at his primary school. He was eight when the family moved house and he had to change schools. Then he began playing up, not listening in class and always claiming that he was too tired to do his homework (there was only a small amount of it), feed his hamster or pick his clothes up from the bathroom floor. It was not, as everyone thought, because of the new school. It was by chance that his father saw Adam going to the toilet in the night. He had always been a good sleeper before this.

Adam's parents found that having to pass water at night had become a regular event and, now they came to notice, he was going to the toilet often in the day. A bladder infection was ruled out by a urine test, but it showed that there was excess glucose. Blood testing confirmed that Adam had diabetes.

IDDM in teenagers

Kirsty was slaving away for her A levels – History, English and French – when she began to lose weight. Half the girls in her class were slimming and so Kirsty was delighted to find that she was successful with minimal effort. She didn't like feeling so thirsty, but she put the tiredness down to all the studying. What upset her was when she began to get some irritation and a creamy vaginal discharge.

Kirsty wanted to be independent from her parents and, although she was tempted to tell her mother about it, she steeled herself to go to the surgery on her own. The discharge was due to a candida infection, which is quite common, but what really struck the doctor was how thin Kirsty had become. She remembered her as a sturdy child. Her first thought was that it was due to anorexia nervosa, but Kirsty wasn't deliberately dieting and the fatigue didn't fit in with this theory. Kirsty had diabetes.

Young adults

If you are in this important age group, your health is your own responsibility. Your mother may still show concern when she sees you, but you are unlikely to take any account of her and you have to be really ill before your friends notice anything wrong.

Freddy was 25, fit and able to hold his own with the best of them at squash. He worked for a computer firm and shared a flat with two other young men. They had a lively social life. The others were surprised when Freddy suddenly became tired all the time, not wanting to stir himself and always ready to get home when they were out on the town. Freddy himself felt drained and he found he was having increasing difficulty in seeing the details on the VDU. He drank a lot – beer, coffee, water – but he never felt his thirst had been quenched.

He had been eating well, but now he began to feel nauseous and to experience vague abdominal pains. As he couldn't face eating, he started to lose weight. After about four days of this he felt so awful that he went along to the Accident and Emergency Department of his local hospital. He hadn't registered with a GP since he had left home. The young doctor found Freddy's heart racing and his blood pressure low. His test proved Freddy had diabetes.

Older adults

IDDM is typically a young person's problem, but not necessarily so.

Amy was 70 – hardly a youngster. Most people tend to put on weight in middle age and lose a little in their seventies and eighties.

25

Amy had never been overweight so she looked quite gaunt when she lost 6 kg (1 stone). She also developed a constant desire for cups of tea and had problems with her water. She had difficulty in getting to the toilet in time, and it was so often.

Her doctor was sympathetic and spoke of stress incontinence, but did not immediately think of diabetes. At Amy's age, he would have expected her to have NIDDM if she was going to have diabetes at all, especially as she'd had an uncle with diabetes who had got by with a change of diet as his only treatment. The urine test did suggest that Amy was diabetic, but it did not seem appropriate to restrict her diet like her uncle. Instead, the doctor started her on an antidiabetic tablet. Amy got worse, but on a regimen of insulin injections twice a day, her weight crept up to 50 kg (8 stone) and she regained control of her water.

If diabetes runs in the family it is likely to be NIDDM, but, in a minority of cases, there is more than one with IDDM. In a few families, both forms of diabetes have turned up. It may be that sometimes non-insulin-dependent diabetes can develop into the insulin-dependent type. It cannot happen the other way, because in IDDM nearly all the insulin-producing cells have been destroyed by the time the illness reveals itself. As in Amy's case, medicines aimed at stimulating these cells cannot work and a change in diet alone may do more harm than good.

NIDDM

NIDDM affects 90 per cent of those with diabetes and is on the up. Most people who develop this type of diabetes are over 30 when they are diagnosed and three-quarters of them are overweight. The classic symptoms of diabetes – thirst, passing unusually large amounts of urine – are often very mild and there is a much lower risk of ketoacidosis, a severe manifestation of diabetes leading to coma.

Unlike IDDM, the illness is partly reversible. If you give insulin to someone with IDDM, their body uses it gratefully. In NIDDM, however, an underlying problem is that the body *cannot* make good use of its own insulin, so giving it more does not help. Some NIDDM sufferers are actually making more insulin than normal, but are still unable to cope with the high levels of sugar in the blood and tissues.

Although NIDDM becomes more prevalent among the older age groups, and is especially common among women with a middle-age spread, it occasionally appears in a young person. This used to be called MODY – maturity onset diabetes in youth. There are some families in which the cause of diabetes is largely genetic and the disorder affects those of all ages – children, adolescents and adults. For most of those who develop NIDDM, as well as genetic susceptibility, there have been many years of an unbalanced diet and sedentary lifestyle.

Back in the eighth century, the Hindus unkindly referred to diabetes as 'a disease of the rich, and one which is brought about by gluttonous overindulgence in oil, flour and sugar'. The English physician Thomas Willis, in the seventeenth century, was more sympathetic. He felt that 'prolonged sorrow' had undermined the diabetics' resistance, allowing them to become ill. Today in the West there is more diabetes and more coronary disease among doctors than the general population. This accords with both the Hindu and Willis' views. Doctors have stressful lives and can afford plenty of meat, fatty and sweet foods at the expense of cheap, healthy vegetables.

Diabetologists in the USA reckon that 2.5 per cent of Americans have NIDDM without knowing that they do. It is masquerading as a kidney, heart or eye problem. Because the diabetic symptoms are so slight, the secondary effects are allowed to develop. It can easily happen that you go for advice about, say, swollen ankles, and the doctor will deal with that problem without considering that an underlying cause could be diabetes.

Douglas went for an insurance examination when he was 58. He understood that he had had a touch of diabetes about ten years ago. He had been given a diet that he had followed for several years. Then he felt well and assumed that he had licked the problem. He had always smoked 20 cigarettes a day, seldom more, and he drank a few pints of beer at the weekends. He had a happy home life and his job in local government was not stressful. No one in the family had ever been diabetic to his knowledge: they had all died of heart and blood pressure conditions.

In the last couple of months, he had been getting unusually puffed and exhausted – for instance, when he did any of the DIY jobs he had always done. He also felt a vaguely unpleasant sensation in his chest – not bad enough to be called a pain – when he had sex these days. The insurance doctor was thorough and spotted signs of artery disease in Douglas' eyes, and the blood test results came back showing diabetes. Meanwhile, a coronary angiogram, a special investigation, showed that the arteries supplying Douglas' heart were slightly narrowed. Douglas is due to have a triple bypass operation and, meanwhile, he has given up smoking, cut down his alcohol intake and started on specific treatment for his diabetes.

Diabetics are especially likely to suffer damage to all three coronary arteries, but usually in the parts that respond well to surgery. It was a plus for Douglas that he did not have high blood pressure as this lessened the risk of his experiencing troublesome eye or kidney complications and of his artery problem, atherosclerosis, worsening.

Cindy was 15 when she was diagnosed as being diabetic. Her grandmother, mother and middle brother, John, all had diabetes. John was three years older than Cindy and had been 14 when he developed it. Her older brother, at this point 20, was so far in the clear. With this family history, everyone thought of diabetes straight away when, after a cold, Cindy seemed to lose all her vitality and even fell asleep when her favourite group were performing. Her mouth and throat felt uncomfortably dry as the cold came on, but it was even worse when the other cold symptoms cleared up.

Cindy's mother had never needed insulin – (she was 52 when Cindy developed diabetes), but managed to stay well with a careful diet and tolbutamide tablets. John had found it more difficult, but his NIDDM was considered to be a family trait. It seems likely that he will need to go onto insulin in the end. Cindy wants to deal with her diabetes by having a super-healthy lifestyle. The modern diabetic diet is much more palatable than when her grandmother first developed diabetes. At that time, almost all carbohydrate was forbidden. Now it is realized that a high-carbohydrate, high-fibre diet with plenty of fruit and vegetables provides the energy that people of Cindy's age must have, while putting the least strain on the metabolism.

A lot of young people these days are vegetarians, so this type of diet was no hardship for Cindy. She also organized her time so that she partook in sport regularly and frequently and she built glucose self-testing into her daily routine.

Other forms of diabetes and related conditions

Gestational diabetes mellitus (GDM)

A positive test for diabetes is done only during pregnancy, usually from the fourth month onwards (see page 69). As this kind of diabetes can harm the developing baby, even if the mother feels fine, screening for GDM is part of routine antenatal care.

Two per cent of pregnant women are found to have GDM and, of these, two in five go on to develop true diabetes within a few years. This is usually of the NIDDM type.

Impaired glucose tolerance (IGT)

With this, there is an excess of sugar in the blood, but not as much as in full-blown diabetes. Nevertheless, there is a 25 per cent risk of its occurring sooner or later. This condition may come to light by chance, when you are having a blood test for some other reason.

Latent diabetes

In some people, the glucose level in the blood goes up abnormally high under conditions of stress, but later subsides. The 'stress' may be an infection or any other severe physical or mental stress. Being overweight is a stress in itself and can also be a factor. Certain medicines, especially steroids, may also throw a strain on the insulin production system (see page 20).

With IGT or latent diabetes, even if you don't develop IDDM or NIDDM, you are at increased risk of atherosclerosis (silting up of the arteries with fat), coronary disease or problems for your newborn baby (see Chapter 7). Although you don't have any symptoms of illness, it is important to have regular checks and, urgently, review your lifestyle. Do you have a healthy diet, are you a healthy weight, do you take regular exercise and not smoke?

Secondary diabetes

Any illness that affects your pancreas – the gland where the insulin cells are – can cause diabetes. Pancreatitis (inflammation of the pancreas) is one such, which may be caused by an infection or long-term overindulgence in alcohol.

Uncommon glandular disorders that may involve the pancreas include Cushing's disorder and acromegaly. Starvation – so-called 'tropical diabetes' – can have a similar effect, and so may some unusual genetic problems, such as hyperlipidaemia (too much fat in the blood), muscular dystrophy, and Huntington's chorea.

Glycosuria (glucose in the urine)

This happens in diabetes or any other condition in which there is extra glucose in the blood. Some people release a flood of glucose into the bloodstream immediately after a meal and this overflows into the urine temporarily. This is a quirk that has no relation to diabetes and does not cause problems.

Similarly, there are other normal, healthy people whose kidneys allow glucose through into the urine even when there is no excess of it in the blood. This is called renal glycosuria ('renal' means to do with the kidneys). Renal glycosuria is commonplace during pregnancy, but it has no long-term effects.

Mike had a fright when he was accepted for a planner's job in the health service, subject to a satisfactory medical. He had answered all the questions on the form with a confident 'No', including those about smoking, psychiatric illness and diabetes, so the on-the-spot urine test showing sugar made him worried that he would look like a liar. Follow-up blood tests let him off the hook, but he had a nerve-racking week, waiting for the results.

That was over ten years ago. He is celebrating his fortieth birthday on Saturday, happy and healthy.

4

Risk factors
and how to minimize them

If possible, you want to avoid having diabetes altogether. What are your chances of never developing this disorder? About 49 to 1, if you take the statistics for the population of Great Britain. However, the proportion of diabetics of both types is increasing, and the risk of your being one of them goes up with your age. Some groups are especially susceptible. For instance, if you are an Asian man of 60 or over the odds are 1 in 4.

What makes a person vulnerable?

First of all, it depends on something over which you have no influence: your parents. Until gene therapy becomes more advanced, perhaps in the twenty-first century, you are stuck with the genes handed down to you in your chromosomes. Every cell in your body contains an identical set of 46 chromosomes that you have inherited. If your chromosome number 6 is different from the norm in one tiny detail, you are prone to develop an autoimmune reaction (see page 23) and, ultimately, IDDM. This only happens in particular circumstances, but, at present, we have only a vague and incomplete idea of what these may be.

In NIDDM, the genetic input is more direct. If both your parents had this disorder, your chances of becoming diabetic would be 3 to 1. Of course, they are much less if only one parent is affected or some other relative, such as a grandparent or aunt. In some people, there is a tie-up between the genes that influence in favour of developing NIDDM and those for obesity.

What action to take

You can't swap your family, but forewarned is forearmed. You will be extra alert to the early indications of diabetes (see Chapter 2) and you can deal with it in the early, relatively harmless stage, cutting short the development of the pernicious secondary effects. There are also ways of avoiding putting unnecessary strain on the insulin-producing beta-cells of your pancreas.

Watch your weight First and foremost, it is important to keep your weight within a safe range (check with the chart on page 118). It is unhealthy to weigh much below the norm and sensible to build up the deficit if so. It is much more likely, however, that you will find yourself a little too heavy or definitely fat. Being overweight – whether you are diabetic or not – makes the insulin in your body less effective. Your pancreas will be called upon to make more of the hormone than usual – an obvious strain on the system.

It is a nuisance, but to ward off NIDDM in particular or to begin treatment if it has already developed, it is essential to go on a reducing regime of diet and exercise (see page 121). Even if you are unlucky enough to carry the obesity genes, they can only make you fat if you eat too much or the wrong foods.

Modify the type of nourishment you have The national diet is unhealthy and leads to more people in Britain suffering lethal heart and artery diseases than in any other country in the world. The same diet increases the risk of diabetes. To avoid such problems, cut down your fat intake and rev up the carbohydrates and fibre. The amount of protein the average person has is probably about right (see chapter 12).

Some carbohydrate foods throw a sudden strain on the pancreas by urgently demanding more insulin. These include sugar-sweetened drinks, sweets, pastries, chocolate, cakes and sweet biscuits, to excess, and sugar sprinkled on fruits and cereals. Even if you are not diabetic, you can experience an unpleasant hypoglycaemic attack. If you have a meal, especially breakfast, consisting of rapidly absorbed carbohydrate foods, such as sugared cereal or white bread and marmalade, or both, your blood sugar may peak and stimulate a flow of insulin. These foods are quickly digested, so your blood sugar soon subsides and there is more insulin that you can use. You are at risk of a shortage of glucose in your blood – hypoglycaemia – which makes you feel queasy, faint, sweaty and shaky.

Although such concentrated sugary foods can leave you temporarily low in glucose, they can still put weight on you. Go easy on this type of food, but, when you do eat it, make sure that you also have something else (such as milk or vegetables,) that take longer to digest, and raise your blood sugar slowly, but for longer.

Dogs, like many other animals, do well on one big meal daily. This does not suit us. We thrive on having not only three meals, but also top-ups in between. That is why employers allow coffee breaks and many of us have a drink and a biscuit before going to bed. Eating small meals often is sensible as it means a steady glucose level and no sudden huge demands for insulin.

Avoid emotional stress This produces an automatic flood of glucose into your blood and can tip the balance towards IDDM. If you suffer a major trauma (one we all experience at some time is a bereavement), you may notice the diabetes-like effect of feeling thirsty. It is almost automatic in Britain to give cups of tea to those who have had an unpleasant shock and maybe this is why.

You can't undo what has happened, but if a disaster strikes, you should try to alleviate the effects as soon as possible. Don't keep a stiff upper lip, but talk about what has happened and your feelings to whoever is available.

After the Aberfan pit disaster, when a number of schoolchildren were killed, an unusually high proportion of their mothers developed the autoimmune type of diabetes (IDDM). Nowadays, an army of counsellors would have been sent in to help, but, at that time, the healing value of talking wasn't recognized.

Avoid long-term tensions and worries They don't have such a dramatic effect in precipitating diabetes as acute stress, but they can make you more *susceptible* to either type. If you are going through a tough time, it is sensible, not soft, to seek help. Counselling may be suitable for the simpler problems or a stress management course may help with business difficulties. Psychotherapy from a qualified clinical psychologist or a psychiatrist can help deeper troubles, while you may need medication in addition if you have slipped into a clinical depression or anxiety state.

If you are frequently tense or a natural worrier, consider asking your GP about relaxation classes: they may help and can do no harm. There is no shame in being sensitive, but it is downright silly to allow stress and tension to undermine your health, including, perhaps, your insulin system.

Viral infections These have a reputation for being possible triggers of autoimmune disorders, including IDDM. We don't know which viruses might be responsible, and there is no inoculation or specific treatment against them, but a healthy lifestyle of regular exercise, fresh air, work and fun and a sensible diet offers some protection against infection.

Any physical illness adds to the burden on your glucose/insulin system. Some have a special relevance. For instance, any disease of the pancreas is likely to upset the beta-cells. Pancreatitis can occur in anyone as a result of an infection, but, more often, it is caused by too much alcohol being taken over a long period. This is an added reason to moderate your drinking. Indications that all is not well with your pancreas include loss of weight, putty-coloured motions and pain in the back.

Pregnancy Chapter 7 is all about this subject, so suffice it to say that this obviously produces an extra load on your insulin requirement and, quite often, this leads to a temporary form of diabetes. It is important to have a blood test partway through pregnancy, even if you feel perfectly well. It is also good sense not to let your weight shoot up too fast – you *don't* need 'to eat for two' when there is a baby on the way! Your metabolism automatically makes the necessary adjustments for you to nourish the baby and you from your normal diet.

Certain genetic and hormonal illnesses The following carry an increased likelihood of developing diabetes:

- overactive thyroid (thyrotoxicosis)
- Cushing's syndrome
- acromegaly
- Down's syndrome.

Medicines that may bring on diabetes The main ones are:

- steroids, like prednisolone
- thiazide water tablets, like frusemide
- antiepileptics, like phenytoin.

What to do when you have diabetes

Most of the advice and risk factors mentioned so far apply even more strongly when you actually have diabetes. There are also other sensible precautions that you should take.

- Always carry a card with information about you, your diabetes, your treatment and a contact. Your diabetes adviser will supply you with a card. It is important. Wear an SOS or Medicalert bracelet or medallion, too, especially if you travel away from home.
- Inform your partner, family, nearest neighbour and work colleagues or teachers about your diabetes and the basic facts about hypoglycaemia, unless you are on a diet-only treatment.
- If you are on insulin or pills, always carry glucose tablets and, preferably, Hypostop gel too, in case you have difficulty in swallowing.
- Carry your insulin on you, which keeps it at the correct temperature.
- Have near at hand always, your automatic finger-pricker and strips for blood tests, for routine and special checks. Keep a diary and record the results, so that you and your doctor can trace any trends.
- Keep to a routine for meals and exercise, as far as possible.
- Be alert for symptoms of a hypo. If you feel slowed down, muddled, sweaty or shaky, if you have a headache or just feel odd, or your heart is thumping, take some glucose, and then decide what to do.
- Every day, do one thing for you – something that isn't concerned with work, diabetes or duty to anyone else.

Practicalities of living with diabetes

Work Almost all occupations are open to you as someone with diabetes, but you will not be accepted for the armed forces, the fire service, the police or to pilot aircraft if you have diabetes when you apply, unless your only treatment is by diet. If you are already working in one of these areas and you are on insulin or tablets, you must tell your employer. Also you must do this if you are in any kind of job in which a lapse of attention – as occurs during a mild hypo – could be dangerous for you and other people. Train or coach driving, driving a heavy goods vehicle or running a signalbox are jobs that are probably out of the question if you are insulin-dependent, but you may be able to negotiate a deal if your diabetes is well controlled by pills.

If you encounter problems with company pension schemes, life insurance or health insurance, ask for advice from the British Diabetic Association (BDA) (for their address and phone number, see the Useful addresses section at the back of the book).

You can work round shifts and canteen meals with a little ingenuity of your own, and there is no reason for you having more sick leave than the next person. Do tell a colleague what to do if you have a hypo and it comes on too quickly for you to do something about it yourself.

Driving Even if you only drive for pleasure, you must tell the DVLA – this is the law. If you are on insulin, you will get a licence for one to three years at a time. On tablets or diet alone, you will get a licence that expires when you are 70 and you then have to reapply. If there is any change in your health, you are duty – and law – bound to inform the DVLA.

Don't drive any vehicle, even a bicycle, for at least a week after starting on insulin or tablets (check with your doctor when this will be OK). Never drive on an empty stomach and have some glucose tablets, biscuits, non-alcoholic drink and your glucose monitoring kit to hand. You are not safe to drive unless your glucose reading is over 6 mmol/l (108 mg/dl). If you feel a hypo coming on, pull over to the kerb or onto the hard shoulder, switch off the engine, take the key out and then have your glucose. Move out of the driving seat to the passenger's side and turn on your hazard warning lights. Wait patiently until you feel better, then check your glucose. Nibble biscuits during the rest of your journey and review the reasons for your having had a hypo when you did.

Motor insurance Unless you tell your insurers about your diabetes, your policy will be invalid and so you will be breaking the law if you drive. Some companies increase the premiums unfairly. You can get advice from the insurance brokers of the BDA. (See the useful addresses section for their address and phone number).

Exercise and sport In general, it is good for you to use your muscles, except in the week or so following any laser treatment to your eyes. Check with your doctor how long you should not take part.

Like anyone else, if you have heart or joint problems, you will be limited, but your diabetes need not hold you back. Because exercise lowers your blood sugar level and makes the insulin in your system more effective, you may need to reduce your dose of insulin before a game by two to four units, and take a snack before or after it. You don't usually need to alter your pill dosage, but you may need to have a snack.

As with food, your body best appreciates regular, moderate amounts of exercise – you just have to go to a little trouble if you want to run a marathon or win at Wimbledon. Pot-holing, hang-gliding and scuba-diving are not advisable and, for other water sports, have a companion. Hypostop glucose gel comes in waterproof bottles, which may be handy if you are liable to be in the water.

Travel You can go anywhere by any form of transport, but you need to be prepared. Take with you:

- diabetic card and bracelet or medallion to inform other people if you are ill or involved in an accident
- letter from your doctor about your diabetes and your treatment, with a summary, if possible, in the language of the country you are visiting (this may save you the hassle of being mistaken for a drug addict because of your syringes and needles)
- medication to cover twice the time you anticipate being away, of either insulin or tablets
- testing kit and diary to note the results
- treatment for hypoglycaemia (glucose tablets and gel, can of soft drink, glucagon-giving kit if you are on insulin)
- foil-wrapped muesli bars, Mars bars and small packs of dry or digestive biscuits for snacks if meals are delayed or don't fit your schedule
- antidiarrhoeal medicine, such as codcine phosphate
- paracetamol for minor aches and pains – *not* aspirin, which may interact with your antidiabetic tablets
- phrase book.

TAKING TO THE AIR Many airlines provide special diabetic meals, which you have to order a week in advance. These are no better for you than the standard airline fare, but less palatable. Either way there is likely to be a little too much fat and not nearly enough starchy food (you can adjust for the latter). About fifty per cent of airlines operating from Britain, say they will provide extra bread rolls with or between meals, but you cannot rely on them. There may also be difficulty in getting a non-alcoholic low-calorie drink and none of the airlines will serve meals at other than their scheduled times.

Tell the stewardess that you are diabetic, so that they can help if you have a hypo. Drink plenty of non-alcoholic fluids. Check you have a supply of plain biscuits and the medication and testing kit described above for any travelling with you.

HOW THEY SAY IT

- In France: Je suis un (une) diabétique; insuline.
- In Germany: Ich bin Diabetiker; insulin.
- In Italy: Sono uno(una) diabetico(a); insulina.
- In Spain: Soy diabético(a); insulina.

Sophy was 24 when her diabetes started. She was on holiday in an idyllic village along the coast from Malaga. At first she blamed the weather and the local water for her raging thirst and having to find a toilet wherever she went. The Spanish doctor tested her urine and from the flood of words she grasped 'diabetica'. She considered going to a town where there might be an English-speaking doctor, but was lucky enough to get a flight home almost at once through her travel insurance. This year, she is equipped with her insulin and all the diabetic kit – and a few relevant phrases.

The British Diabetic Association (BDA)

Joining the Association, or its equivalent in the USA, Canada or Australia, is the single best precaution you can take against problems to do with diabetes because of:

- the sense of belonging to a club or community as it has 130,000 members and 400 local branches
- up-to-date, authoritative answers it gives to all your questions concerning diabetes, by post or via the Care Line
- the latest news on research that is relevant to your health and treatment, as well as recipes, articles and information about events are brought together in *Balance*, its bimonthly journal.

For the addresses and telephone numbers of the BDA and other organizations see the Useful addresses section at the back of the book.

5

Treatment

If you have just learned that you or someone close to you has diabetes, you may feel devastated, but take heart. There is well-tried, effective treatment available and, straddling the world, there is a network of dedicated researchers working on your behalf. Every day they are acquiring a greater understanding of this complicated disorder and developing better ways of dealing with it.

At present, there are three types of treatment: diet, tablets and injections. More than half of those who have recently been diagnosed can control their diabetes satisfactorily by means of a change of diet alone. Of the rest, 20 to 30 per cent also need antidiabetic medicines by mouth, while the same percentage require insulin, which has to be given by injection. You can work out roughly which treatment is likely to be best for you:

- if you are under 40, you are almost certain to have IDDM and to need insulin, plus a diet that enables you to reach and maintain a normal weight
- if you are over 40 and overweight, you definitely need a low-calorie diet and maybe also an antidiabetic medicine. Metformin (Glucophage, Orabet) is helpful if you are slimming, but is unsuitable if you are pregnant, fond of alcohol, have other health problems or are feeling your age
- if you are over 40 and slim or average weight, you may only need a diet to keep your weight steady, but you are likely to need antidiabetic tablets as well (there is a wide choice); a minority may need insulin, and although most of this group has NIDDM, some have long-term IDDM.

The basic aims of treatment

These are:
- to restore the metabolism to as near normal as possible
- to prevent or reverse any secondary ill-effects:
  - keeping the blood sugar within bounds reduces damage to the

39

small blood vessels and through them, the eyes, kidneys and nerves
- avoiding excess fat in the blood lessens the risk of atherosclerosis, high blood pressure and heart attacks. ✓
  ref

The treatments for IDDM

By definition, this *must* include insulin otherwise as Charles II's doctor said of another patient, '. . . he will waste away, grow weak, fall into sleep and die'. It wasn't until 1921 that two young men in Toronto, realizing that diabetes was a hormone-deficiency disease, decided to make an effective extract of insulin from animal pancreas glands. Nowadays there are not only beef and pork insulins but a human preparation. This does not come from dead people, but, by means of genetic engineering, certain bacteria have been made to produce human-type insulin.

Insulin is supplied in two formulations.

1 *A clear, quick-acting solution* This starts to act within half an hour of the injection and is effective for four to six hours. It deals with the influx of glucose into the bloodstream after a meal, if taken 20 minutes beforehand. Some people use it regularly in this way. It is also the preparation of choice in an emergency situation.
2 *A cloudy, delayed-action solution* It takes effect in 4 to 6 hours and continues for 8 to 14 hours. There is also an extra-slow form – ultralente – with a duration of 24 to 36 hours.

These figures apply to the beef and pork insulins; the action of the human type begins and ends sooner. Although you would imagine that the human insulin must be the best, it does not suit all diabetics, and some tend to get too many hypos that catch them by surprise.

How and when to take insulin

It's like buying a new outfit. There is a wide choice and it is a matter of what suits you as an individual.

A common pattern is to take a dose of both clear and cloudy insulin twice a day, before breakfast and before supper.

Syringes and needles are disposable, but you must take care that neither children nor drug addicts can get hold of the used ones, nor that anyone else can be accidentally pricked by them.

Insulin pens are a neat way of dosing yourself as they are easy to carry and easy to use, especially if you want to give yourself injections before every meal.

Insulin pumps, which provide a continuous supply, were thought to be a wonderful breakthrough a few years ago. In fact, though, they proved clumsy and troublesome, requiring intensive supervision because of frequent swings into ketoacidosis and, less often, hypoglycaemia.

Choice of regimen

There are three levels of care to choose from: minimal, average and intensive.

Minimal care

Zoë, an uncooperative 16-year old fell into this category. She was too busy growing up to bother about her diabetes. She went along with the diet, more or less, although, as she didn't want to put on weight, she sometimes cut down on the carbohydrate.

To save herself any bother, she tried taking all her insulin once a day, before breakfast, with an evening dose if she felt she needed it – and it was convenient. The trouble was that she often took exercise on the spur of the moment and alcohol when there was a party. This meant that she frequently landed in an exercise- or alcohol-induced hypo. In the latter case, or when she was experimenting with cannabis, she was not always alert enough to detect the early signs of a hypo. On other days, Zoë might have a typical adolescent lazy time, listening to music. These were also times when she might unthinkingly or defiantly indulge in chocolate.

Despite difficult days, Zoë managed to get by at school and socially, and she played down her frequent trips to the toilet and drinks of diet coke.

When she bothered to do them, Zoë's blood tests often showed a glucose level of around 16 mmol/l before meals. Her urine was frequently positive for glucose with an occasional plus for ketones.

If she continued in this way, Zoe's health would be on the line and she would run the risk of eye, kidney and artery problems in the years ahead. If she had been younger her growth would have been impaired. As an adolescent, her body has an extra resistance to insulin and there is no way that a once-a-day dose of it can be effective. Only for very elderly diabetics with the NIDDM type of diabetes is a once-daily regimen adequate.

Average care

Sean was older, 32, and more level-headed than Zoë. He was a solicitor, married, with one child.

He chose the twice-daily routine of the clear and cloudy insulins, and an extra dose of the quick-acting type at midday if he was taking a client to lunch. He felt well and had no symptoms of thirst or passing too much water. He might have a mild, manageable hypo up to once a week, but rarely a severe attack. His blood glucose was usually between 8 and 11 mmol/l before meals and his urine showed sugar now and again, but never ketones.

Sean is managing his diabetes rather better than half of all those with IDDM. If he had been younger his growth would not have been affected. Nevertheless, the DCCT ten year survey has shown conclusively that tighter control of glucose levels than that achieved by Sean at present would increase his life expectancy and greatly reduce the chances of long-term complications of diabetes occurring.

Intensive care

Veronica was a physiotherapist and particularly comfortable with things medical. She invested all her energies into everything that she undertook, which was excellent for her patients. She was also a perfectionist. She had been diabetic for three years, since she was 23, and had conscientiously established a three-times-a-day insulin routine. She seemed very fit, but when her specialist suggested that she might like to try the so-called 'ideal' regime for diabetics she agreed enthusiastically.

It involved intensive self-monitoring (see page 10) with frequent blood tests and urine examinations to guide her on the optimum dosage of insulin in relation to her food intake and activity. The aim was to keep her glucose down to between 6 and 7 mmol/l before meals, just above the value for non-diabetics. Her urine would then always be negative for sugar and keytones. Because she was often on the brink of a hypo – for instance if lunch was late or work had been particularly physically stressful or energetic – Veronica found she had to test her blood glucose four times a day, and at odd times if she felt uneasy.

She was always adjusting the dosage, but, in general, she managed with a multidose pattern (MDI). She took clear insulin before each of the three main meals, plus the slow-acting form first thing and at bedtime. Of course, she followed the dietary advice precisely, breaking her nourishment down into six sessions, which meant having three snacks between her three usual meals.

This was five years ago. After nearly 18 months of following the 'ideal' regime during which time she felt that her whole life was dominated by dealing with her diabetes, she became less obsessive and the detailed routine became more automatic. There is not the slightest sign of any diabetic damage in Veronica's eyes, nor indeed anywhere else. Her uncle, who had the same type of diabetes, died at 51 of a coronary. He had also been a smoker.

Injection technique

As an adult, you will be taught the technique of injecting yourself the first or second time you see your specialist, and you will be supervised until you are proficient at it. The best areas for the injections are your upper arms and thighs or your abdomen, but you must use a different spot each time.

It feels most comfortable if the insulin is at room or body temperature, which will happen automatically if you carry it around with you, especially if you use an insulin pen.

Unless you are very dirty, there is no need to cleanse your skin. If you must, use soap and water and rinse the soap off, but do not clean the area with alcohol or spirit as it hardens the skin and tends to make the injection sting.

When you are ready, pinch up a fold of skin and push the needle in quickly, at a shallow angle so that it goes through the skin, but not into the muscle underneath. Then inject the insulin, count to three, quickly withdraw the needle and press the place with your finger for a few moments.

Young children should receive their injections from someone who is experienced at it, so that they don't feel any discomfort and are not frightened. To distract a child from thinking about whether or not the injection will hurt, and as a step towards taking control later, it is good for them to give a favourite teddy an injection at the same time.

Occasionally, a small child may be allowed, as a 'grown-up' treat, to give themselves their injection. From the age of ten onwards, children may be encouraged, but never pressurized, to start doing their injections themselves. By the age of 14, most of them will have taken the job over altogether.

Monitoring technique

This is the other special technique you must learn as a diabetic. Fundamental is the estimation of the amount of glucose in your blood, using a drop of blood from your finger or, with the help of a mirror, your ear lobe.

First, wash your hand – or ear – in warm water, rinse off the soap and dry with a clean towel. Make sure your hand is warm before you start.

Use the automatic finger-pricker, and if the blood doesn't ooze out readily, massage your finger towards the tip. Next, use the colour-change strip according to the directions (you must have a watch to time the test). Finally, compare the colour with the standard chart.

Glucose biosensors have made home-monitoring even easier. They provide a digital display of the reading of your blood glucose within 30 seconds.

How often should you test? Two tests a day is the minimum if you are to keep your diet and insulin dosage on track – if your diabetes is already stabilized. Doing four tests a day is better (one before breakfast, one at lunch, one at supper and one at bedtime). If the results are satisfactory, you need only repeat the extra tests on alternate days. You may need to test at other times, too, – say, before and after unaccustomed exercise, during an illness or if you feel ill and don't know why.

Urine testing This gives limited information, but is a useful, easy extra check.

A colour-change strip is held in the stream of urine and, after waiting the recommended time, the colour produced is compared with the chart on the bottle. Urine tests give an indirect idea of the amount of glucose in the blood if a positive result is not due to a quirk of the kidneys.

You can also test for ketones in the urine, using a similar method. This is the only practical way of detecting their presence and can be a vital warning that ketoacidosis is coming on. Otherwise, you may not realize, if you are feeling nauseous or vaguely off colour, that you are in danger of this serious development occurring (see page 73).

Using your monitoring Monitoring means taking control of your diabetes, rather than being the helpless victim of the illness.

The way you use the information from the blood and urine tests can help you in three respects:

- to avoid or cut short a hypo (you need food or glucose straight away if your blood sugar is at or below 4 mmol/l; see page 81)
- to avoid or get help urgently, for the serious condition of ketoacidosis (see page 73)
- to fine-tune your diabetes care or warn you your control is failing badly.

The rule of thumb to remember when you are interpreting your glucose level is that food and stress make it go up, while exercise and insulin – or a delayed meal – push it down. One high glucose reading when you know you have eaten more than you should is a signal to give yourself an extra 1 to 4 units of clear, quick-acting insulin. Then, check your glucose again in two to three hours time. If it is 18 mmol/l or less and you feel OK, don't worry. If the glucose is going up past 19 mmol/l, however, and especially if you don't feel well, give yourself another 4 to 8 units of fast-track insulin and check your urine for ketones. More than one plus shows that you are seriously short of insulin and should contact your diabetic adviser. If you start vomiting, you must get to a doctor or a hospital as soon as possible.

If you have a rising blood glucose-level, but no ketones in your urine and you are feeling well, or if you just have a persistently high glucose level, it means that the dose of insulin you are on isn't enough to deal with what you are eating. If you are overweight, you need to cut down your intake or adjust the balance of fats, carbohydrates and protein. If your weight is normal, you may need to adjust your dose of insulin upwards by steps of 1 to 4 units. Get advice from your doctor or diabetic nurse.

Diet

Chapter 12 is all about this subject, but it is important to mention it here, too. Diet is the other essential of treatment. You can't get away with ignoring your diet and hoping that the insulin alone will restore your metabolism to normal and keep you healthy indefinitely. With IDDM, you will probably have lost weight and strength, so your first task is to rebuild the tissues, including muscle, that your body had to burn as fuel when it couldn't cope with carbohydrates. When you have reached a weight you feel happy with (check with the table on page 118), all you have to do is to maintain it with a well-balanced mix of foods.

A balanced diet is what top nutritionists recommend in Britain, America, Japan and Australia for *everyone*. Too many in the developed world die of heart disease and strokes and have their later years marred by atherosclerosis and blood-pressure problems. Those of us with diabetes of either type are especially vulnerable to them, but there is something we can do. The right diet is the best preventative treatment and, as a bonus, it also provides some insurance against cancer. You may be young enough to feel that all these illnesses are remote from your situation, nothing to do with you, but why not get the best out of life at *all* stages? This includes getting the best nourishment.

Guidelines for a maintenance diet
- *For 15 to 20-year-olds*
- *female*   29–33 kcal per kg of your ideal weight, daily (1 kg is about 2 lbs)
- *male*   33–40 kcal per kg of your ideal weight.
- *For 21 to 55-year-olds of either sex*
- *physically active* 31–35 kcal per kg of your ideal weight
- *mainly sedentary* 22–26 kcal per kg of your ideal weight
- *pregnant*   in the first 3 months, 26–35 kcal per kg of your ideal weight
                   in the last 6 months, 29–37 kcal per kg of your ideal weight.
- *For those over 55 or overweight* – 22 kcal per kg of your ideal weight.

It works out like this:
- if you are 15 to 20 and your ideal weight is 47.5 kg (7½ stone), you will need 1,350 to 1,550 kcal per day if you are female, 1,550 to 1,880 kcal if you are male
- if you are 21 to 55, whichever your sex, and should from your height weigh around 57 kg (9 st), you will need 1,770 to 2,000 kcal daily if you lead an active life – or 1,250 to 1,480 kcal otherwise
- if you are pregnant and the clinic says you should weigh around 57 kg (9 st) in the first 3 months, you need 1,480 to 1,650 kcal per day;

if you are in the last six months of pregnancy and around 66.5kg (10½ st), is about right for you, you need 1,914 to 2,450 kcal daily
• if you are over 55 or overweight and ought to be about 66.5 kg (10½ st), 1,450 kcal per day is enough to keep you at the same weight.

Whatever the calorie count, your day's nourishment should be divided up like this:
• *carbohydrates* 50 to 60 per cent (the average intake in the UK is 46 per cent)
• *protein* 12 per cent (most people consume between 10 and 15 per cent)
• *fat* 30 per cent (the average is 46 per cent).

About 15 years ago, it was thought that carbohydrates were harmful to diabetics and should be cut down as far as possible. All the diabetic associations in the world now agree that this is nonsense. Diabetics, like other people, need to step up their carbohydrate intake.

The most beneficial kinds are bread, rice, pasta, potatoes and other vegetables and fruit. The ones to avoid are those that give you a sudden, large dose of sugar, such as jam, marmalade, honey, syrup, sugar, fizzy drinks, sweets, chocolate and cakes. Keep these as treats, not for every day.

The big class of nutrients to watch and almost certaintly to cut down are the fats – butter, oil, spreads, ghee, cheese, full-cream milk and its products and red meat. Pastries, cakes, sweet biscuits and chocolate need to be restricted not so much because of the amount of sugar they contain but the fat. It is probably worthwhile to shift from animal fats to polyunsaturates, such as corn, sunflower and fish oils, and the monounsaturate, olive oil. Even then, though, you still need to limit the quantity.

A general point: it is better to be a nibbler than a gorger if you are diabetic. If you have three, medium-sized meals, plus three snacks in between, this evens out your glucose level through the day and is a safeguard against hypos.

The fourth ingredient in a good diet is *fibre*. It comes in two forms:

• insoluble, which you find in wholemeal, wheat bran, breakfast cereals, brown rice and jacket potatoes
• soluble, which is found in peas, beans, lentils, oats, fresh and dried fruit, and the gum guar which can be taken in sachets or granules to

reduce glucose absorption. You can buy guar from pharmacies and health shops.

There is no need to bother with commercial preparations since there are so many foods that supply fibre naturally.

Fibre is valuable, not because it is nourishing, but because it:

- improves glucose metabolism, so that you don't have peaks or excessive blood levels (the soluble type achieves this)
- reduces the level of cholesterol and other fats in the blood (the soluble type does this)
- reduces the risk of colon disorders, from constipation to cancer (the insoluble type has this effect).

Increase your intake of fibre gradually and be sure to drink plenty of water to enable you to digest it. You should also check your blood glucose, as you may need a lower dose of insulin.

Now you have the groundwork, you need to make a meal plan with the help of a dietician. Considerations are:

- your food preferences (check back over the last week to remind yourself what you enjoy)
- your schedule, including times of meals and where you will be
- timing of periods of physical exercise.

For the best results in terms of glucose control, try to be consistent in your eating. Multiple injections or an insulin pump give you a little more leeway, but your body thrives on a regular rhythm in food intake as in everything.

When you have an off-colour day and you don't feel like eating, as all of us with IDDM experience now and again, you must continue to have at least some insulin and some carbohydrate. Fruit juices, jellies and soups, in several little meals, may go down most easily.

Hypoglycaemia The commonest causes are:

- a delayed meal
- unaccustomed exercise
- taking alcohol on an empty stomach
- oversleeping more than three-quarters of an hour.

To avoid a hypo, you may reduce your dose of insulin by 10 per cent before playing sport or have a carbohydrate snack. For more on this subject, see below and page 77.

HYPO SAVERS
To take immediately when you feel the symptoms:

* Lucozade or similar
* glucose tablets, preferably with water
* glucose gel
* plain biscuits
* jam
* sugar lumps
* sweets.

Follow up this immediate supply with one of these:

* digestive biscuits or chocolate.

The fat delays the absorption of the glucose, so the effect is slower but lasts longer.

Alcohol Viv got the job! The interview had gone well, despite that awful question: 'What do you consider are your main weaknesses?' She was to start in the New Year.

Sally and Brian were waiting for her in the Paviour's bar to hear the news. She enjoyed a cool glass of low-sugar lager, and their congratulations, before getting into her Mini to go home, a little later than usual.

She lost concentration at the second set of lights and went through a red light – under the noses of two policemen. When they stopped her, they noticed that her speech was slurred and there was alcohol on her breath. Viv realized she was going into a hypo and stuffed the dextrose tablets she had in her handbag into her mouth. She felt better very quickly, but the police and the rest of the affair took weeks to sort out.

The disadvantage of specially modified drinks – usually lagers – is that if one aspect is improved, another may be made worse. The low-alcohol lagers contain more sugar than normal, while the low-sugar types, such as the one Viv chose, have more alcohol. Alcohol inhibits the liver from releasing glucose when the blood level is low when, for instance, a meal is delayed.

You don't have to be teetotal if you have IDDM, but you may upset your carefully managed metabolism if you drink more than two units at a sitting, three times a week.

The treatments for NIDDM

Diet

While insulin is an absolute must in IDDM, diet is central to the treatment of NIDDM. In fact, modifying your diet may be the only thing you need to do to keep it under control. In NIDDM the diabetic symptoms of thirst and needing to go to the toilet frequently are often mild and so curing them is a relatively easy matter. The major aim of your treatment is the prevention of serious complications – a greater risk in this type of diabetes than in the insulin-dependent type.

None of us – fat or thin, diabetic or not – can eat and drink whatever we like. Most of us would be barrel-shaped in no time if we did. Nevertheless, it is frustrating to feel restricted when it comes to the simple pleasures of food and drink. They are an integral part of family life, friendship, celebration and comfort. It takes strength of character, commitment and cooperation over diet to make the difference between success and failure. Success means long-term health and being able to live a normal life.

Most of us are already over our ideal weight by the time we become diabetic. Health is then added to the factors of fashion and appearance as incentives for losing weight. The first essential is to cut down the calories. This has an immediate beneficial effect: your blood glucose level goes down. It is healthy to work towards achieving your ideal weight at any stage, but the sooner you start, the more responsive your body and your diabetes will be.

If you mean to lose weight, you must aim at an intake of 1,000 calories daily, or less but then under supervision. To mark time at any particular weight, you can reckon on using 30 to 35 kcals per kg (2 lbs) of your body weight, depending on how physically active you are. This works out at 1,700 to 2,000 kcals daily if you weigh 57 kg (9 st), 1,950 to 2,300 kcals if you weigh 66.5 kg (10½ stone), or 2,250 to 2,600 kcals if you weigh 76 kg (12 stone) or more. Any cutting down *must* be gradual.

You will find calorie counts for all the recipes in diabetic cookbooks and in many others, as well as those given in women's magazines. While counting calories is a tiresome chore to start with, it soon becomes second nature. You will also be able to make adjustments when you go to a restaurant or have a take-away meal.

Saeed, at 58, was a happy man. He loved his food, his family and the grocery shop they ran together. Being in the food business, there was never any shortage of good things to eat in the home – unlike the hard times he had endured as a boy. His wife and daughters liked cooking for him.

It was a shock, and very unwelcome news, when he was told that the painful boil on the back of his neck was due to diabetes and that he had high blood pressure into the bargain. The final blow was to hear that 89 kg (14 stone) was far too much for a man of 1.7 m (5 ft 7 in) and that he must go on a diet straight away.

The traditional Asian diet includes plenty of vegetables, beans and fruit with carbohydrates in the form of rice, chapatis, nan and poppadums, but Saeed had a sweet tooth. He couldn't resist jalabi, kulfi, gur and chocolate, and he liked his food cooked with plenty of ghee or oil. Fried samosas were a special favourite of his. Particularly because of his blood pressure, Saeed also had to cut down on salt.

His whole family wanted to help, so they all cut out sweets except for special occasions, left out added salt in cooked dishes and changed to brown rice and wholemeal chapatis. They had more whole dahl, guar, bindi, karela and sweetcorn for the sake of the valuable – and filling – fibre of the skins. Red meat was kept to a maximum of five times a week, with dahl, fish and chicken as replacement.

Saeed is slowly losing his big stomach and his wife and daughters are pleased that they, too, are slimmer.

The 'whole family' approach is essential if a child is involved, but it is good sense for any family to review their eating habits if one member is overweight or diabetic.

Once you have taken off some weight, you need to work out a diet that is palatable and satisfying and will keep the weight off. Exercising on a regular basis helps and the more you exercise, the less severely you have to restrict your eating.

Antidiabetic tablets

If you are overweight and over 40 when you develop NIDDM and your fasting glucose level comes down to 7.7 mmol/l or less with a change of diet, that is all the treatment you need. However, dieting may not be enough. If your fasting glucose level (measured first thing in the morning) consistently tops 11 mmol/l or you still have symptoms, you probably need to take antidiabetic tablets. This is *as well as*, *not instead of*, your diet.

These tablets stimulate the cells in your pancreas to make more insulin. There is a range of tablets, but they come in only two chemical types:

* Sulphonylureas:
  - chlorpropamide (Diabinese), which was the first to be developed, is very long-acting, which can be troublesome if the dose is set too high and you experience a hypo
  - glibenclamide (Daonil) is the one in most common use and is fairly long-acting; hypos occur in one in three users
  - gliclazide (Diamicron) is similar to glibenclamide, but becoming increasingly popular as it is thought to reduce the risk of blood vessel complications; hypoglycaemia is less likely than with glibenclamide
  - tolbutamide (Rastinon) is short-acting and safer with a hypo, especially in older people
  - glipizide (Glibenese) is short-acting; the smaller tablets are easier to swallow than tolbutamide ones
* Biguanidines:
  - metformin is the only one now in use and is unsuitable for heavy drinkers and those with kidney, liver, heart or lung disorders; it has the advantage of reducing the appetite in those who need to lose weight; you have to take it *with* or *after* a meal, not *before*.

Neither sulphonylureas nor biguanidines are suitable in pregnancy or when breast feeding.

Kenna was only a few pounds overweight when she was diagnosed diabetic after a run of urinary infections. She was only 42 and, although she kept quite well to the recommended diet, her glucose level never settled within the acceptable range. Diet alone often seems to work best for older and overweight sufferers. Kenna was started on glibenclamide – the standard treatment – but, instead of feeling better, she kept getting headaches, couldn't concentrate at work and felt weak. She was constantly teetering on the edge of hypoglycaemia. Although she felt better after a sweet drink and a biscuit, it all began again the next day.

Rather than juggle with the dosage of the long-acting glibenclamide, Kenna's doctor substituted the short-acting drug glipizide, twice daily. She has had no further trouble.

Bonus There are no prescription charges for these drugs.

The side-effects The main side-effect is hypoglycaemia, but, occasionally, there are rashes, digestive and bowel upsets or flushing when you drink any alcohol.

Clashing with other medicines Some antibiotics (but not penicillin-type ones), ibuprofen, phenylbutazone, aspirin, warfarin, beta-blockers, MAOIs and probenecid may cause problems.

Blood tests

Even if you don't need tablets, it is important to check your glucose level regularly, although you won't need to do this as frequently as those with IDDM need to. You doctor will make routine checks, but if you get the knack of doing the tests yourself (see page 44), you are more independent. You can check your blood sugar anywhere and any time, which is especially useful at times of stress or during an illness – or if you feel off colour and don't know why. Testing is important as the results warn you if your blood glucose is creeping up and sneakily undermining your health.

Some people prefer to make do with the old-fashioned urine tests to monitor their diabetes (see page 44). They are a lot better than nothing, but are not very accurate.

Insulin in NIDDM

Most of us with NIDDM can control our diabetes with diet and tablets if not diet alone, but a minority need to switch to insulin to achieve this. It can be because the pancreatic cells are no longer capable of responding to the tablets or, for some reason, the diet keeps slipping. Whatever the cause, though, if your blood glucose level stays high, the answer must be insulin. You will probably need to take it only once a day, but when you are on insulin, you will have to get used to testing your blood to avoid hypos.

If you are overweight, even insulin cannot work as well as it should, so make a new resolution to lose some weight. You don't need to lose much to make a big difference.

See Chapter 12 for more on diet.

6

Diabetes and Sex

Nothing affects a person's self-esteem as much as the feeling that there is something wrong with them sexually. As you could expect, with a disorder that impinges on the nourishment of every cell of the body, diabetes can affect the smooth working of the sexual systems of both men and women.

The effects of diabetes on women

In general, there is nothing to worry about if you are a woman and have diabetes – except that you are likely to be fully fertile and so cannot take chances with contraceptive precautions if you don't want to become pregnant just now.

If a girl develops diabetes of the IDDM type before the usual age of puberty, her periods will often start later than the average. The younger the girl at the onset of diabetes, the longer this delay is likely to be. This only means an extra year or two without the hassle of periods, but to an adolescent growing up, it may be upsetting if her body doesn't behave exactly like those of the other girls at school.

Added to this, the changing levels of the sex and growth hormones at this sensitive age often make it difficult to control the diabetes. Glucose values shoot up and down and a teenager may not always comply with the rules for managing her diabetes.

Charlie – Charlotte – was 14¾ when she had her first period, and it wasn't even plain sailing then. Her periods seemed to arrive at any old time, which was annoying and sometimes embarrassing. It was no wonder that she was moodier and more irritable than most adolescents when she was coming up to her GCSEs. It didn't help matters that there was a good deal of family conflict at the time – her parents were revving up for their divorce. It wasn't that they didn't care about Charlie, but they were preoccupied with their own emotional troubles. Charlie's diabetes became wildly unstable and she had a run of hair-raising hypos, which her doctor suspected were due to her playing around with her insulin dosage.

So-called 'idiopathic' (which means the doctors don't know the cause of it) brittle diabetes almost always crops up in adolescent girls – often those who are slightly overweight and experiencing family problems. Some of them go on to develop psychosomatic disorders, such as anorexia or bulimia, or an emotional condition of anxiety or depression (see Chapter 11). This makes it more difficult than usual to stabilize the glucose levels, which means an increased risk of diabetic damage to the eyes or kidneys.

In Charlie's case, the home situation calmed down when her father finally left, and she had the good fortune to find a boyfriend who was intelligent and concerned. His support and gratifyingly good results in her exams gave Charlie's self-esteem the lift it needed. She no longer tried to attract her mother's attention by using her illness, but set her mind on the future. For this she had to achieve control of her diabetes.

As a woman with IDDM, you may find that your menstrual cycle is always a little irregular, and you may need to adjust your dosage of insulin during the time of your period. Around 20 per cent of women have to raise the dose a few units during the first two days, and a few need a good deal more. Another 10 per cent require a *decrease* in the run-up to a period, which is difficult to judge if your cycle is haphazard. It means testing regularly. It is useful to have someone knowledgeable, for instance a diabetology nurse, to discuss these matters with.

These changes in insulin requirement are probably directly due to the hormonal fluctuations at this time, but some of us feel especially hungry for carbohydrates – sweet ones – before a period is due. A few diabetic women, by contrast, feel slightly nauseated then and so eat less than usual.

The enjoyment of sex

This and the capacity to respond are in no way diminished by diabetes, unless there has been damage to the nerves (diabetic neuropathy). Even then, any adverse effects on sex – for instance, being too dry – are rare. Also, for the years when most people are most sexually active, it has been shown that those with IDDM have no more problems with sex than anyone else. If you have NIDDM, you may have less confidence in yourself in bed, which may partly be because of being overweight. This is one thing you can do someting about – with courage and determination. If you can cope with diabetes, you can certainly get your weight down if you set your mind to it. The bonus is that doing so is good for your general health, too. You need the tenderness and the security of feeling that you are loved, and your physiology will respond as it should.

If you are careless about your health and diet schedules, having NIDDM makes you extra susceptible to infections of the urinary and sexual organs. Candida (thrush) in the vagina is common because the yeast that causes it thrives on sugar. If you have this problem, you need to take your diabetes in hand, as well as using the creams and pessaries your doctor will prescribe.

Urinary infections, such as cystitis, can also be troublesome if diabetes isn't strictly controlled. The treatment is with antibiotics: several are available.

Your fertility

When insulin first came in, no-one knew how to use it in the best way and many diabetic women were in such low health that they didn't have periods and even more had difficulty in conceiving. This is not the situation today. You may have irregular periods, but you are as fertile as anyone else, so be careful.

Contraception It is perfectly safe for you to go through a pregnancy if you are diabetic, unless you have serious kidney or heart disease. If you have eye problems, they must be dealt with before you decide to have a baby.

As for all women, pregnancy is best when it is planned. As a diabetic, it is especially important that you prepare for it thoughtfully and learn something about the possible complications. Meanwhile, you need contraception, of whichever type fits the bill for you. It is essential to discuss the choice fully with your GP or, better still, to go to a Family Planning Clinic.

If you take no precautions, you stand an 80 per cent chance of becoming pregnant within a year. There is a 10 per cent chance if you rely on a condom or a diaphragm, and much worse odds with spermicides or the rhythm method. Worst of all is withdrawal. Even with an IUD, you run a 4 per cent risk of pregnancy, as well as the likelihood of heavy periods and the danger of infection that can accompany this method of contraception. The Billings method of natural family planning has not been assessed in diabetic women, but it is difficult for most couples to abide by the long periods of abstinence required.

For most women with diabetes, the Pill is the most effective and the easiest to manage method of contraception. The type containing a high dose of oestrogen worsens diabetes, but the newer low-dose combined Pills are suitable for you if you are a young woman with IDDM, free from eye or kidney problems. If you have NIDDM and are overweight, or if your blood pressure is a little high, the Pill is not for you.

Progestogen-only Pills are actually less safe for your diabetes than the low-dose combined types, and also slightly less effective. But most failures with the Pill are due to forgetting a dose or gastro-enteritis washing it out.

Low-dose and progestogen-only Pills may produce irregular periods or them stopping altogether. They usually start up again, though, as soon as you stop taking the Pill.

Progestogen implants can be inserted under the skin and, if necessary, removed. Long-acting injections of the hormones do not allow you this flexibility – you cannot undo them if they don't suit you or if, after all, you want to start a family.

The other certain methods of contraception are surgical and permanent; sterilization for the woman or vasectomy for her partner. Most women want to retain the option of having a child unless they are seriously ill. With modern methods of managing pregnancy, diabetes doesn't undermine your chances of motherhood. You have only to stop your contraceptive and, sooner or later, you will become pregnant. (See the next chapter for more on pregnancy.)

The effects of diabetes on men

While diabetic women today have few problems with sexual performance and fertility, it is a more complicated matter for the man. The male sexual apparatus involves several nerve mechanisms. The central features are the erection – the enlargement and hardening of the penis for long enough to complete the act – and the release of the seminal fluid, which carries the sperm. The whole process is set off by a surge of emotion at the sight or touch of the right partner. It happens automatically, unless the man makes a conscious effort to suppress the response.

The automatic or *autonomic* nervous system operates under its own control and takes over during sex. It has two branches – the parasympathetic and the sympathetic. They work in conjunction to make the sexual act possible. The parasympathetic produces the erection by manipulating the blood supply to the penis, and the sympathetic branch causes the ejection of the semen from its storage vesicles.

It is amazing that all this happens with precise timing and sequencing in such a light-hearted atmosphere most of the time. But problems arise in some diabetic men. They are a minority, but still a significant number. About a third of diabetic men are impotent, that is they cannot achieve an effective erection. There are three areas in the nervous system where a fault can occur to spoil the satisfying experience of intercourse. They are in the brain, the parasympathetic and the sympathetic parts of the nervous system.

Psychological difficulties

These are particularly common among diabetic men.

Gerry was 23. He'd had diabetes since he was 11 and felt himself to be an expert in self-monitoring his blood glucose and fine-tuning his diet, activity and dosage of insulin. Of course, he made occasional slips, but his control was generally good.

When he fell in love for the third time with a beautiful girl called Candy, he was sure that she was the one. He had had no particular difficulties with sex up until this time, when it mattered so much to him. He knew that diabetes sometimes caused impotence and this preyed on his mind.

He found it was very hit and miss as to whether or not he could maintain an erection and when he did manage to, he ejaculated far too soon. It was a disaster and getting worse.

Electrophysiological and hormone tests results were normal. Gerry wasn't an alcoholic and he wasn't on any of the medicines that can interfere with autonomic functioning, but, to relax himself with Candy he would often smoke some cannabis and this proved to be part of the problem. Cannabis, like excess alcohol, can cause impotence. In Gerry's case, there was also a psychological aspect. His anxiety caused the premature ejaculation, but, more fundamentally, Gerry had convinced himself that he was a sexual no-hoper. His self-esteem had touched rock bottom.

The doctor reassured him and told him to stop smoking cannabis, but it was Candy's patience and cooperation that helped him the most. Sex now works out fine for them on the majority of occasions.

The psychological factor is probably the most important of the three discussed here. Sex is closely bound up with your emotions and, for men in particular, it can easily be blown off course by anxiety, depression or loss of confidence. If you have any hint of a night or morning erection, that is a hopeful physical sign and it would be well worth checking out your psychological state. Unless your family doctor has an unusual leaning to psychiatry, you should ask to see a psychiatrist who has special expertise in the interplay between physical symptoms and emotional problems.

Sex is a game for two, so your partner should be brought into the picture. Sexual difficulties can undermine a partnership and lead to disagreements and misunderstandings. If your problem is largely psychological, expert help and support with a shared approach stands a good chance of success.

Parasympathetic neuropathy

Diabetic damage – that is, the effect of too much glucose in the blood – can upset the parasympathetic system and interfere with the erection mechanism.

Sympathetic neuropathy

This can lead to a failure to ejaculate, which, obviously causes infertility as the semen isn't released.

In most cases, the sympathetic and parasympathetic branches are both affected.

Autonomic neuropathy In up to 40 per cent of diabetes sufferers, the autonomic nervous system doesn't function at 100 per cent efficiency, but has not been damaged permanently. Indications that the autonomic system is impaired are more likely to show up in those over 40 and in anyone who has had diabetes for more than 20 years. The symptoms are often vague and not what you'd expect. For instance, you might experience momentary giddiness when getting up, because of low blood pressure; diarrhoea, inconveniently at night; or a curious absence of sweating of the legs and feet, but drenching sweats of the upper part of the body. This latter sometimes comes on just after a meal. Also, bladder problems, such as a very slow stream, may also be due to autonomic impairment, but they are not usually an early sign. Eye and kidney problems, too, may, in part, be the result of autonomic nerve damage.

Those with IDDM and those with NIDDM are equally susceptible to autonomic problems. This indicates that the harm is done by high glucose levels rather than hypos, which occur mainly with IDDM. This, in turn, means that exercising more care in keeping the blood glucose in check should improve matters. The logic of this line of thought has been found to be true in practice. So, if, after testing, your sexual difficulty is seen to have originated from faulty autonomic input, the first essential step you can take is to tighten up your control of your blood sugar level.

Other causes of male sexual difficulties

Factors that may confuse the issue include poor control of blood glucose levels, drinking too much alcohol, being overweight and being older, say 50 onwards.

Impotent men frequently have eye problems, another indication of less than perfect diabetic control. For these cases, there is no special cure, but potency can return if the man is willing to cut down on alcohol and high-fat foods and be more meticulous about testing himself and adjusting things accordingly.

Numerous medicines can interfere with sexual functioning – especially those used to treat psychological disorders, such as depression and anxiety. Others are the drugs used to lower blood pressure, including beta-blockers, steroids, used in many conditions, and salbutamol, the stand-by for those suffering chest problems. You need to check with your doctor about whether or not a new medicine will have side-effects on your sexual system whenever it is prescribed.

Occasionally, you may have difficulties with sexual performance because of a shortfall in the male hormone, testosterone. As hormone treatment doesn't work, if the testosterone level is low, the best approach is to boost your allover physical condition. To do this you need exercise, fresh air, a healthy diet whether you are taking insulin or not, regular checks of your blood sugar – and mental stimulus. Always have something to look forward to: 'treats' don't have to be big and costly, just enjoyable.

If you have a definite physical block on performing sexually, all is not lost. There is a range of treatments you may like to consider. They need to be explained and discussed with a sexologist (a medical specialist in the subject). Possibilities include:

• Ericaid, which is an expensive device that applies suction to the penis to make it enlarge, with a band applied to the base of the organ to prevent it relaxing too soon

- injections, which you learn to give yourself, into the base of the penis when you want to have sex; may produce erections that last about two hours
- surgical insertion into the penis of an inflatable or a permanently rigid rod (it is wise to try the other methods before going for surgery).

For many couples, particularly for the female partner, the most meaningful and enjoyable part of making love is the closeness, tenderness and touching. Penetration is an extra that may not be worth the effort of the last three ploys mentioned above. They do not enhance fertility, but, luckily, most men with serious problems are in the older age groups where it is less likely that they will be wanting to father a baby.

7

Pregnancy, birth and the baby

So, you want to start a family. No matter how many other women have managed it, this will be your own unique, personal miracle. Because it is such an important step, it makes good sense to plan ahead, prepare for it and find out some essential facts. If you are already pregnant, or suspect you may be, you have some catching up to do.

Genetics

We hear a lot about genes these days and, as a responsible, caring parent-to-be, you will want to know what you may be handing on to your child through your genes, the blueprint for his or her development.

The good news is that there is almost never an occasion when doctors would advise a diabetic woman or man to hold back from having children on genetic grounds. Even if your child does develop diabetes later, it is something they can live with – after all, you do. During this century, medical research has taken much of the sting out of diabetes, and it is discovering new facts all the time. There is work currently being done that is looking into the possibilities of preventing the disorder altogether, nipping it in the bud before it has done any damage, and, of course, better methods of dealing with it have become established.

Even if you or your partner is diabetic, the chances of your child developing the problem are probably much smaller than you think.

If you have IDDM

The risk that your child will develop it later is:

- 1 per cent chance if you are the mother
- 6 per cent chance if you are the father
- 30 per cent chance if you are both diabetic.

So, at the worst, the odds are against your child being affected.

If you already have a child with IDDM, the chances of a brother or sister having it are, on average, 8 per cent. They are higher if blood tests show that the baby has antibodies against its own insulin-producing cells. This is evidence of a propensity to an autoimmune reaction, which is when the body's defence system turns against part of itself.

With identical twins, there is a 35 per cent chance that both will develop diabetes if one does. Even so, the risk is less than 50:50.

All this can only mean that there must be other factors involved as well as the genes.

If you have NIDDM

The risk that your child will develop it is:

- 15 per cent (6 to 1 against) if either parent is diabetic
- 75 per cent if both parents are diabetic.

If you have one child who has NIDDM (which is less likely before the age of thirty), there is a 10 per cent chance that any brother or sister will develop it in due course. In the case of identical twins, either *both* are likely to be diabetic or *neither* will be.

If you have the rare form of NIDDM, sometimes called MODY

There is a different, stronger genetic tie-up known as autosomal dominant. Your child will have a 50 per cent chance of developing it, and the risk is the same if your partner or the child's brother or sister has this type of NIDDM. It can come on at any time from early childhood onwards, but commonly does so when people are in their thirties. Unlike IDDM, insulin is not necessary for several years after the start of the illness.

Preparing to be a parent

Before insulin came to be used in the 1920s, the chances of a woman with diabetes becoming pregnant were minute. After all, the only treatment was near starvation. If, by some miracle, a woman managed to conceive and get through the pregnancy, she only stood half a chance of surviving the birth and the baby was almost certain to die.

What a different story it is now! Diabetic mothers are at scarcely any greater risk than other women. This is partly because of insulin, but also because of the use of blood tests, which are much more accurate than those used on urine, and the realization of how important it is to the baby to control the mother's blood glucose throughout the nine months of pregnancy.

If possible, take stock before you become pregnant. Pregnancy gives your metabolism a substantial jolt, so prepare in advance, by:

- getting your blood sugar level down to as near normal as possible
- cutting out cigarettes and alcohol
- having your eyes examined and, if there is a problem in the retina, getting it dealt with first.

Preliminary discussions at the surgery or clinic

These should cover the following points:

- as pregnancy makes your system more reactive to carbohydrates, so that your blood sugar tends to shoot up after meals, you will need advice about increasing your insulin to compensate
- if you have had any eye, kidney, heart or blood pressure problems, they will need to be checked as they are liable to worsen if your blood glucose creeps up
- because your baby may be bigger than average, you are more likely to need a Caesarean birth, which means you need to give careful thought to where you will have your baby
- your baby will be at slightly greater risk of developing problems around the time of birth, but the risk can be minimized by keeping to the guidelines given below during pregnancy, and if excellent paediatric care is available in a well-equipped hospital (essential for the newborn of a diabetic mother)

Guidelines for a healthy pregnancy

- Have regular antenatal checks – weekly, fortnightly or monthly, according to your circumstances.
- Carry out blood glucose tests at home up to six times a day, keeping a record to discuss with your nurse or doctor. Learn to adjust your own diet and insulin dosage as necessary meanwhile.
- Have two insulin injections daily, and be prepared to have up to four if control is slipping.
- Do not smoke or drink alcohol for the whole of your pregnancy.

- you will need help and support from your partner, especially in the later stages of pregnancy and after the baby is born, while your body and your diabetes are readjusting – to the excitement and a new lifestyle as much as anything else.

The father should be brought into the discussions from the beginning, but if he is supportive, he wouldn't want to miss out anyway.

Antenatal visits

These are especially important for you and your baby, to prevent anything going off course. Assessment includes an ordinary physical examination, including blood pressure, urine tests for infection and kidney function, blood tests for a range of vital chemicals apart from glucose and, of course, measuring your weight. It is healthy to put on around 11 kg ($1\frac{3}{4}$ stone), during the pregnancy, most of it in the second half.

The size and development of the baby will be assessed by means of ultrasound examinations. If you haven't had them before, don't worry. It is rather soothing when the nurse or doctor slides the sound camera over your abdomen, which has been anointed with baby oil to enable it to slide easily. The result is a moving picture in black and white. You will be given a 'still' of one of the later films to keep.

In the first three months, all the ultrasound reveals is the size of the foetus in relation to your dates, but, by the seventeenth week, the main organs will have formed and a detailed examination is made. Two or three weeks later, the baby's heart can clearly be seen, beating steadily. From then on, it is mainly a matter of measuring how fast the baby is growing. If you want to know, it is sometimes possible to make out the baby's sex from the pictures.

Hypos

The down side of trying to keep your glucose level really low is an increased risk of having a hypo (see page 77). Other people at home need to know the signs and what they need to do to help if one happens. At the first hint, you must take four dextrose tablets, a small bar of chocolate or half a glass of a glucose drink. Always have supplies at hand, but don't take more than one of those suggested.

Your partner, or whoever is likeliest to be around, must know the drill if you have got to the point when you can't swallow. Emergency tactics that anyone can adopt are to smear jam inside your cheeks or squeeze Hypostop gel between your teeth. Whoever is with you overnight should know how to give you a glucagon injection in case you have a hypo then. Home treatment must *not* be delayed, even if an ambulance has been called for a severe hypo.

Diet

This may be a nuisance to you during pregnancy – a time when women characteristically develop odd cravings for or aversions to food. It is especially tiresome, even though it is quite natural, to feel extra hungry and to have to struggle to keep your blood sugar in line.

Nadine had the opposite problem. She had always been beanpole thin and endlessly energetic. Now she felt vaguely nauseated most of the time and vomited once or twice, even though she had eaten hardly anything. The doctor thought it might be the standard iron and folate tablets that were upsetting her, so she stopped taking them and tried to eat the right foods to make up for them. She had All-Bran, peas, meat, eggs and wholemeal bread and pasta to supply the iron and fresh, dark green vegetables and cauliflower to supply the folate. At a weight of 55 kg (8½ stone), and 1.7 m (5 ft 7 in) tall, she needed 2,000 kcals a day, which worked out at 30 to 35 kcals per kg of body weight. Nadine found that she managed to eat enough by taking six small meals a day, that is breakfast, lunch and tea, with bigger than average midmorning, midafternoon and evening snacks. Even then, she wasn't gaining weight, so Jake, her husband, insisted that she should switch to part-time work and have a day-time rest. Even as a secretary, sitting down, she was burning up calories more than twice as fast as when she was resting. When she got into the swing of having more leisure time, she relaxed and her weight inched up. The pregnancy went ahead well, and her baby daughter weighed 3,350 g at birth – perfect.

The final hurdle

If everything goes well, you will go into labour and have a normal-sized, full-term, beautiful baby within a week either way of the date you have ringed in your diary. In some cases, however – for instance, if your blood pressure is nudging up or the baby isn't getting enough nourishment via the placenta – the birth may be induced a week or two before the baby is due. This is to ensure the safety of you and your baby.

You can expect to have a vaginal delivery as a rule, but there are some circumstances in which it is safer to have a Caesarian birth. These are not confined to mothers with diabetes. They are when:

- the mother has a small pelvis
- the baby is big
- the baby is lying in an awkward position
- the placenta is in the way.

It is difficult, even with ultrasound, to judge the relative sizes of the baby and the birth canal. If in doubt, your obstetrician may prefer to do a pre-planned Caesarian, rather than put you and the baby through a stressful test. If you have a Caesarian birth, you are likely to have an epidural anaesthetic as this is safest for the baby and then you don't miss the experience of those first precious moments of your baby's life in the outside world.

During the birth, it is important to keep your blood sugar spot on. If it is too high, the baby is at risk of having a hypo as soon as he or she is born, so you may be given an infusion of glucose and insulin during the critical period.

As soon as the baby has been born and the afterbirth – the now-redundant placenta – has been delivered, your insulin requirement drops sharply, so you will soon be back to your pre-pregnancy dose.

As an insurance, your baby will receive special attention in the first few hours after birth, but, usually, you can expect to go home as soon as any other new mother and baby. About 20 per cent of babies born of diabetic mothers have a brief fall in blood sugar soon after they are born, so checks are made. Usually, a prompt feed puts matters right, but a glucose infusion can be given if necessary.

What to do if you have other forms of diabetes

Brittle diabetes If you have this type of diabetes it is almost impossible to stabilize (see page 114), so you stand a greater risk of experiencing problems during pregnancy or in labour. Vomiting or blood pressure that gets too high can make your diabetes worse. It means treading a tightrope of testing and adjusting your dose and your diet, but there is the reward of your baby to look forward to.

Gestational diabetes mellitus (GDM) Everyone, diabetic or not, has urine tests at the antenatal clinic. As one of the effects of pregnancy is that the kidneys allow some glucose to pass through, a urine test indicating the prescence of sugar means very little. A high *blood* sugar result on more than one occasion in a woman who isn't diabetic, however, sets alarm bells ringing.

Normally, a mother-to-be has to produce more insulin than usual, because of the effect of some hormones released by the placenta, the baby's nourishment system. If you happen to be predisposed to diabetes through your genes (perhaps you have a relative with either IDDM or NIDDM), your insulin-manufacturing cells may not be up to meeting the increased demand. A shortfall of insulin lets the glucose level mount in your blood and then you have GDM. Your baby is extremely sensitive to an overload of glucose.

Fiona wasn't diabetic, although she knew something about it because her mother was. When the diagnosis had been made, two years before, Fiona's mother had been 53 and rather overweight. She had gone to the doctor for a check-up and a slimming diet. She had been feeling increasingly tired and put it down to her middle-aged spread. A general examination, plus urine, then blood tests showed that she had a high blood sugar level. She was diabetic. So far, by rigid adherence to the diet prescribed, she had lost some weight and avoided the need to take pills.

Fiona was 28 and perhaps a little overweight when she became pregnant. She felt perfectly well and there were no adverse results from tests during the first three months. So, it came as a shock when the clinic doctor told her that she had rather a lot of sugar in her urine and that she would have to have a special blood test – a glucose tolerance test (see page 7). At the end of the test, her glucose level was 13mmol/l; 9 mmol/l is the upper limit of the normal range. She had developed GDM.

She was anxious lest the baby might have been affected, but, by the time GDM usually arises – around the fourth month – the baby's organs are formed and all that is left is for them to grow. Too much glucose from the mother at this stage would tend to make the baby too big, involving difficulties with the birth. However, at four months it is not too late to avoid this by bringing the mother's blood sugar down to near normal. It is common practice in antenatal clinics to test all mothers-to-be for GDM at the twenty-eighth week, in plenty of time to correct matters.

Fiona had put on rather more weight than most of the other mothers and, as soon as the diagnosis of GDM was made, she was advised to restrict her diet. She was allowed 1,600 kcals a day, with no sweet, fizzy drinks, cakes, sweets or sweet biscuits. It proved impossible for Fiona to keep to this, as she had an insistent appetite and felt that she should be allowed to eat as much as other pregnant mothers.

The pills for NIDDM, which Fiona's mother may have to take in due course, are not safe to take in pregnancy. Fiona was disappointed to find that she had got to have insulin injections twice a day. She started off with a small dose of isophane, a medium-acting type, but this had to be increased several times. It levelled out at the thirty-second week, and she cheered herself up by thinking that it wouldn't be for much longer.

She went into labour 48 hours ahead of her due date and young James was born some 6 hours later – lovable, perfect and weighing a comfortable 3.4 kg (nearly $7\frac{1}{2}$ lbs). He took his first feed well and hasn't looked back since. Fiona's labour and the follow-up period (the puerperium) were supervised as if she were an established diabetic. After the birth, her glucose level was tested several times, but it rapidly returned to normal.

Fiona is not a diabetic, but she *is* watching her weight as a sensible way of reducing the chances of her developing the disorder later or at least delaying its onset. The risk is quite high in her case – about 50 per cent – and Fiona is likely to develop GDM whenever she is pregnant again. In future, she will be tested for GDM from the beginning, as she may develop it earlier next time. If GDM isn't treated, the baby has an increased chance of becoming diabetic as an adult, as well as the other effects of being exposed to excess sugar.

Pregnancy is no big danger for diabetic mothers, the person most at risk is the foetus. That is why it is vital to take every precaution and put up with any restrictions.

Breast feeding

You don't have to miss sharing this unique experience with your baby just because you are diabetic. The composition of your milk will be precisely right and it will confer on your baby the same protection from infection as any other mother's milk. Of course, it means taking a little extra care with your tests and your diet and you will need between 25 and 50 g (1 and 2 oz) more carbohydrate daily than usual, but this is worth doing.

The effects on the baby

The outlook for babies born of diabetic mothers has improved dramatically since the 1970s in the industrialized world. In England and Wales, if the mothers have attended specialist diabetic centres, the perinatal mortality rate (that is, the number of babies who die around the time of their birth) is almost down to the same low figure as that for non-diabetic mothers. The sad thing is that in the few cases where babies have been damaged, nearly always this could have been avoided.

The commonest cause of serious trouble for the baby is its mother's blood sugar being far too high during the pregnancy – something that can be corrected, so long as you test for it. High glucose, and also high blood pressure, interferes with the blood supply to the placenta – the baby's lifeline. It supplies vital oxygen as well as nourishment to the baby, and no one can live without oxygen.

The other serious problem is disruption of the baby's normal development during the early weeks. If there is very variable control of the diabetes, especially if the mother also smokes and drinks, this poses the main danger to the unborn baby. Again, this is in your hands, and timing is crucial. By the twelfth week, the foetus is still very small, a few inches long but, already, he or she is recognizably a little human being. By the fiftieth day after conception, the baby's heart is working, and three weeks later all the main organs have been formed. You have to start protecting and looking after this precious new life you have created from the time you start making love without using contraceptives.

The main feature of the last six months of pregnancy is the baby's phenomenal growth. If your blood sugar is allowed to creep up during this time, the result is an outsize baby, one that is longer, heavier and, like an overfed child, with more fat than healthy, firm tissue. Bigger does not mean better for babies and an obvious disadvantage is that the birth will be slower and more stressful for both of you! It may well be safer to have a Caesarian delivery.

If you are diabetic, your baby's first few hours are critical. The respiratory distress syndrome, where the baby has difficulty with its breathing, crops up in nearly one in five of those born ahead of their due dates, from $36\frac{1}{2}$ to $38\frac{1}{2}$ weeks. The underlying cause is likely to be the mother's high blood sugar – something that can be avoided in many cases.

Of otherwise healthy babies, 20 per cent develop mild hypoglycaemia if their mothers are diabetic. During the sojourn in the womb, the baby's system has been used to providing enough insulin to deal with the extra-generous supply of glucose received via the placenta. As soon as the cord is cut, so is the excess sugar supply, but it may take a little time for the baby to adjust the insulin production. The hypo it experiences isn't usually serious and doesn't last more than a few hours, but it underlines the importance of trying to keep your blood sugar as near normal as possible during labour. This is a medical problem. It is your doctor's responsibility to check your baby's blood sugar several times during the first six hours. The baby may be given glucose by a tube into the stomach or intravenously if he or she doesn't take enough in the first feed.

Later development

Studies have not shown any long-term effects on mental development of being born to a mother with diabetes. The only physical result is a 1 per cent risk of developing IDDM by the age of 25.

Jeremy is one of the other 99. When he was born – 44 years ago – diabetes was as dangerous in England as it is in Kenya today. His mother was ill, on-and-off, during her pregnancy and it was thought that Jeremy's chances of survival were slim. He was a big baby – 4.5 kg (10 lbs). He looked strapping enough, but his blood glucose was less than 2 mmol/l and he wasn't interested in taking a feed. The paediatrician wasted no time in getting some glucose into him. It is harmful for the brain to be short of glucose for long, but clearly Jeremy suffered no damage: he is Professor of Neurology at a prestigious teaching hospital, having chosen the most intellectually demanding specialty in medicine, and, in his spare time, he is an able musician. Also, he doesn't have diabetes.

8

Emergency and acute complications

It's useful in everyday life to know what to do if a fuse blows, but also when it is best to call in an electrician. It is much the same with diabetes. You can't expect your body to work harmoniously non-stop with never a hiccup throughout your life. Now and again you may run into a problem, and it is handy to be able to recognize what has gone wrong and what you need to do about it. It is also useful to know how you can avoid similar trouble in the future or at least minimize the chances of its happening again.

Complications – the problems associated with diabetes – are of two types:

- emergency or acute, calling for instant action
- long-term or chronic, requiring long-term adjustments.

This chapter is about the former, which can occur in both forms of diabetes. They are more *frequent* in the IDDM type but can be more *serious* in older NIDDM sufferers.

Ketoacidosis

This is the most dangerous complication of diabetes. Before 1923, it was invariably fatal, but now we have both the insulin and the know-how to beat it. It is also cropping up less often, probably because people with diabetes are so skilled at managing the disorder.

What it is

Ketoacidosis is diabetes galloping out of control, with the metabolism turned upside down by a lack of insulin. Sometimes it is set off by a physical illness, such as a severe infection or a mild heart attack, sometimes because of a muddle in managing insulin dosage, exercise and diet, but, more often, there is no obvious trigger.

> Helen's situation was different again. There wasn't a trigger and, anyway, she wasn't a diabetic. At least that was what she thought.

73

No one in the family had the disorder, so there was no reason for her to think about it. With hindsight, perhaps it was significant that she had to go to the toilet more often than anyone else in the office. At the time, she put it down to drinking a lot: she was always ready for tea, coffee or a coke. She was 23, looked good, felt good and was happy with her boyfriend, Jason.

Then it all started to change. Over a matter of days, all her energy seemed to drain away and she didn't fancy eating – not even chocolate, which was one of her favourites. Her face was flushed and she couldn't put her make-up on smoothly, but it was when she couldn't see properly and her tummy hurt all over that she became frightened. Jason dialled 999 for an ambulance. The moment the paramedics came into the room they sniffed the air. The older one asked if Helen was a diabetic.

Helen was sick on the way to the hospital and began breathing in an unusual way, with big, deep sighing breaths. Her breath smelled peculiar – somewhere between rotten apples and nail varnish remover. The Accident and Emergency Department had been alerted to her condition by radiophone, so the staff were waiting for her.

By the time she got there she was becoming drowsy and a little incoherent, but immediate testing of her blood and urine with reagent strips showed high levels of sugar and also of ketone bodies.

A larger sample of blood was taken for detailed analysis, but the basic treatment was started urgently, without waiting for the lab results. Fluid was dripped into a vein in Helen's arm to replenish her dehydrated state, with insulin to make up the drastic shortfall in her own supplies. Her progress was monitored continually.

The effect of the treatment was miraculous. When Jason visited her the next day, Helen was back to her usual, jokey self. She could hardly believe that she had been seriously ill the day before, but it was an even greater bolt from the blue to learn that she had diabetes.

Of course, they asked her about her previous health and any illnesses in the family. Helen was surprised that the doctor was so interested when she mentioned her Aunt Sonia's vitiligo, the skin condition where parts of it lose their pigment.

What had happened to Helen to throw her metabolism so alarmingly out of gear? She had developed the autoimmune type of diabetes, IDDM (see page 23). Gradually, the cells that produced Helen's insulin had been disabled and killed off by her own defence system attacking these vital cells as though they were invading germs. Other autoimmune disorders include rheumatoid arthritis and vitiligo, so Helen's aunt's trouble gave a hint that there was a tendency in the family for the immune system to malfunction in one way or another.

When Helen's worsening shortage of insulin reached a critical point, her blood sugar rocketed. Her body made an emergency response, which only made matters worse – stimulating the production of glucose and also ketone bodies. Ketones have a characteristic smell. They are strongly acidic, devastating to the normal working of the body. Without insulin the body cannot get rid of either excess sugar or ketones, although it tries to do so through the urine and in the breath, which is what the paramedics noticed when they came into Helen's room.

Helen had most of the symptoms of ketoacidosis, apart from cramps in the legs. She probably didn't worry about the sharp loss of weight because, like most young women, she was always trying to be slimmer. Some sufferers run a high temperature, but in others it is subnormal. Sometimes the rhythm of the heart is disrupted, but this is usually a symptom in older people.

Recognizing when ketoacidosis may be starting to develop is all you can be expected to do. That and getting help, if at all possible, before you are overtaken by deepening drowsiness, running into coma. The precise diagnosis and the treatment given, of course, must be left to the doctors.

Richard was one of Jason's more enthusiastic drinking friends, and they were going to the same stag party. Richard was fairly tanked up when they met. He'd been drinking all afternoon and hadn't bothered to eat anything since a cup of coffee in the morning. Naturally, the drinks at the party showed their effect on him sooner than on the others.

Around midnight, he said he had a stomachache and he was sick. After that he became increasingly stupid and was difficult to rouse. It was Jason, with his recent experience with Helen, who identified the sinister smell of acetone on his friend's boozy breath. He felt like an expert when he explained to the ambulance people that he thought Richard needed urgent hospital treatment for diabetic ketoacidosis.

Richard *did* have ketoacidosis, with much the same symptoms as Helen, but there was no excess glucose in his blood – in fact, very little was found. He was not diabetic; it was an overload of alcohol, combined with a shortage of carbohydrate food, that had sent his metabolism haywire.

Diabetic non-ketotic hyperosmolar coma

Most diabetic ketoacidosis crops up in the first half of life, but it can also occur when you are middle-aged or elderly. Sometimes in this group there is an extremely high blood sugar level and all the indications of ketoacidosis – without the ketones. This is diabetic non-ketotic hyperosmolar coma, the run up to which is impaired consciousness.

This complication can creep up on you without the tell-tale warning odour, and what makes it even more sneaky is that in two out of three cases, it is the very first evidence of diabetes.

Gladys was 63 and still worked in the one remaining baker's shop in the town. She was a favourite with the customers and knew them all. She was what used to be called a 'comfortable body', which meant she was friendly and moderately overweight.

When she went to her GP, feeling the need for a tonic, he was not surprised to find that Gladys' blood pressure was higher than it should be. He advised her to diet, but who could, where she worked? He also prescribed some tablets to bring her blood pressure down – a beta-blocker and a water tablet. This is a mild, standard treatment.

Gladys didn't feel any better. She was just as tired as before and now it seemed that she was passing water all the time. She presumed that was what the water tablets were meant to do. She also found she was having difficulty in concentrating and sometimes gave a customer the wrong number of rolls or the wrong change.

It was after she had been on the tablets for a week and a half that she had a mild fit, which started with her left arm twitching. She went off into what seemed a heavy sleep afterwards.

The doctor thought Gladys may have had a stroke, as he knew she wasn't epileptic or an alcoholic. A blood test at the hospital showed a glucose level of over 50 mmol/l. A urine test would also have shown excess sugar, but Gladys was in no state to give a sample. The treatment she was given was similar to that given to Helen when she had ketoacidosis. It comprised fluids and insulin, plus correction of any chemical deficits found in the blood.

Gladys recovered, but grumbled dreadfully when she was told that she had diabetes and the regime for managing it was explained to her.

In fact, she was lucky. The episode she had suffered could have ended much more seriously.

This type of illness is often triggered by a urinary or chest infection or by medication for another condition. Gladys' blood pressure drugs were the likely cause in her case. Others that may also lead to the problem include cimetidine, steroids, and phenytoin. Sweet, fizzy drinks can be the final straw.

Lactic acidosis

This is similar to the illness just described, but is rare in diabetes nowadays. Occasionally it can be precipitated by the antidiabetic medicine, metformin (Glucophage), so this is best replaced by one of the other preparations, such as tolbutamide or glipizide after your sixtieth birthday (see page 52).

In the early 1970s lactic acidosis arose too frequently, almost always in those using an antidiabetic called phenformin. This was withdrawn in 1977.

Hypoglycaemic episodes

These are the 'hypos' that every diabetic on insulin knows about and wants to avoid. More than a third of those with IDDM suffer a serious hypo at least once, while for 10 per cent, they happen about once a year. An unlucky 3 per cent have their lives messed up by frequent attacks.

The cause

There is a mismatch between medication, food and exercise. The medicine in question is usually insulin, although a hypo can occur when a sulphonylurea antidiabetic drug is being taken for NIDDM. A simple increase in the dosage of insulin doesn't lead to a hypo by itself – there have to be other adverse circumstances. Nine times out of ten it is down to carelessness – having too little food or too long a gap since the last meal or suddenly taking an unaccustomed amount of exercise or going far too long without a break for nourishment.

Risky situations

- the 'honeymoon' period, when you have recently started using insulin. Your requirement for it goes down, but only temporarily. It is a matter of monitoring your blood sugar often until it stabilizes
- the first few hours after having a baby
- if you have lost 3 kg ($\frac{1}{2}$ stone) or more, whether planned or not – if you want to slim, take advice and do it under supervision
- when breastfeeding, if you don't take enough extra carbohydrates (see page 70).
- when, in some women, the need for insulin goes down during their periods
- when you travel and if it is difficult to get your usual diet (airline meals are notoriously short on carbohydrate, so take your own supply of biscuits or chocolate)
- problems in the last three months of pregnancy
- when you have an underactive thyroid – you feel cold and sluggish
- when there is a change in the type of insulin you use (most diabetics today are using human insulin, but anyone on an animal preparation must be vigilant about their blood sugar and the dosage when changing over)
- when girls have eating disorders – anorexia or bulimia nervosa – and have crazy diets and devious ways of getting rid of the food in their bodies, it can be disastrous if they are also diabetic
- when adolescents who are going through a difficult stage, often involving family conflict, deliberately play around with their insulin.

Kim was 17 and on battle terms with her mother. Mrs James had been fussy and overprotective ever since the divorce. For Kim, bringing on a hypo – usually by missing a meal – was the equivalent of getting drunk. She enjoyed the light-headed feeling and she could be as rude and awkward as she liked. No one would blame her – she was 'ill'. Her mother was gratifyingly panicked every time. Of course, in time, Kim matured emotionally and gave up her silly games, but not before she had developed eye problems, which required laser treatment.

Edward's situation was different. He had learned a satisfactory regime for coping with his diabetes long ago. He didn't even need to think about it. He had enjoyed his student years – not studying too hard, nor playing much sport, but listening to music and talking endlessly with his friends.

After he'd scraped through his BSc exams, getting a 2:2, he was lucky enough to find just the job he wanted. He became research assistant in the agricultural branch of a pharmaceutical company. As a junior, much of his work was hands on, with the plants. It involved much more physical activity than in his three relaxed years at university, but he stuck to the same diet and dosage of insulin; they had become second nature.

What had previously been a happy balance was now skewed by his increased muscular output and, on a particularly busy day, he had his first real hypo. He recognized what it was because at the clinic he attended there was a policy with young, healthy patients of allowing their blood sugar to go down to around 2 mmol/l under supervision. This is the level at which most people develop noticeable symptoms.

Edward found the tatty pack of dextrose tablets he had carried about in his pocket for so long for just this situation. He took four tablets and, within minutes, he was feeling better. In the discussion at the clinic later, the cause of the hypo was identified as being the additional exercise involved in his job. Edward has increased his carbohydrate intake on working days.

Hypoglycaemia may be acute, with obvious effects that must be dealt with promptly, or it can be very slight, but continue over a long period. The latter is most likely in older people.

The symptoms and signs of acute hypoglycaemia

These alter with the blood glucose level.

- *3.0 mmol/l* This is the so-called 'twilight zone' when you are not quite on the ball. You can do ordinary tasks, like making the bed, but you can't weigh things up and make sensible decisions or do complicated calculations. It is likely that your nearest and dearest or your workmates will notice the subtle changes before you do.
- *2 mmol/l* Now you may begin to feel and act as though you are tipsy. Some people even become aggressive. You will certainly notice some of the following tell-tale signs:
  - trembling

- sweating
- thumping heart
- hunger
- blurred vision
- mouth dry or overly full of saliva
- dizziness
- headache
- weakness
- pins and needles anywhere

Other people will notice that you look pale, sweaty and exhausted, and your doctor would find that your pulse is rapid and emphatic.

• *Special people*:
  – a child with a hypo may behave badly, sulk, be bad-tempered or have a temper tantrum
  – an older person may act as though he or she is teetering on the edge of a stroke, seeming confused and unsteady.

With so many indications, a hypo doesn't usually get beyond the 2 mmol/l stage because action is taken to reverse it, either by the victim or someone who has been forewarned and knows what to do. When it does progress further, however, this is what happens.

• *1 mmol/l or worse* You are likely to slip into unconsciousness, perhaps with convulsions. Someone else must get some glucose into you (see page 82).

Unawareness of hypoglycaemia Sometimes the symptoms are so mild that you don't react to their important messages. This can happen in long-established diabetics, those taking beta-blockers or those in the early stages of pregnancy. In a few it can happen, ironically, because they are super-conscientious about their diabetes.

Stella was 19 and had been diagnosed as diabetic only a few months ago. She was a perfectionist and, encouraged by her father, she kept her blood sugar under very tight control. Her motto was, if in doubt, increase the insulin or cut out some carbohydrate. The result was that she was so often running with a blood sugar just below normal that her body didn't react as vigorously as others' would when the level became harmfully low. She didn't receive the warnings in the early stages of a hypo on the day she decided to skip lunch so as to get to a lecture at another college. She meant to make up with a big snack at the 3.30 pm break.

At first, everyone thought Stella had fallen asleep during the talk, as she slid down in her seat. When it was obvious that she was ill, one sharp-eyed colleague saw the silver bracelet on her wrist, saying that she was a diabetic on insulin. The college doctor dealt with the situation quickly and efficiently. After this scary episode, Stella – and her father – took a more relaxed and realistic attitude towards the degree of blood sugar control to aim for.

It is a matter of balancing the advantages and disadvantages. To cut out the symptoms of diabetes itself and avoid either hypos or ketoacidosis, you need to try and stay within the 3 to 12 mmol/l blood glucose band. This may be too wide to insure against long-term complications, though, for which a range of 3 to 8 mmol/l is safer. But, remember, from 3 mmol/l down, subtle early mental impairments begin to develop. You cannot guarantee a completely unchanging blood sugar level whatever you do; it's like trying to make the sea lie flat. First, the rate at which your body absorbs the dose of insulin varies enormously from one day to the next. Secondly, if you succeed in keeping your blood sugar level at the lower end of the range, there is the uneasy thought that a hypo may occur in the night. For older people in particular, who may be insulin-resistant, there are health snags in habitually having a little too much insulin in the blood. It is bad for the arteries. The watchwords in all these are reasonable care and flexibility.

What to do if you have a hypo

If you feel that a hypo may be coming on – your concentration is slipping or you start to be a bit of a butter fingers – check your blood glucose, if it is convenient and you feel up to it. It should be 3 mmol/l plus. If the reading is too low or it is awkward to do a test for one reason or another, act now. If you have them, take about four dextrose (glucose) tablets, washed down with water or any other drink to hand. A couple of boiled sweets or sweet biscuits or three sugar lumps or a spoonful of jam will do instead. Glucose, in tablets or as a drink, works quickest, but ordinary sugar (sucrose) is almost as effective.

A friend or work colleague or your partner must know what the signs of a hypo are and be prepared to insist that you take whichever preparation is available, even if you are complaining that you don't

81

want it. If you are drowsy but able to swallow and take a drink, your friend may be able to 'post' the tablets into your mouth.

If that isn't feasible or there is a danger you might choke, the emergency treatment is for them to smear jam inside your cheek or squeeze Hypostop gel between your teeth and then massage your cheek from the outside. A 1 mg glucagon injection into muscle or just under the skin is useful, but its effectiveness depends on your helper's having been trained in the technique (see page 43).

Recovery is usually magically rapid and complete. Afterwards, there must be an analysis of what went wrong. Hypos are unpleasant and can be dangerous, so you want to avoid them in future.

The symptoms and signs of chronic hypoglycaemia

A long-term deficiency of glucose in the blood is not as likely nor as obvious as the acute type, but it can arise in someone taking just a little too much insulin or someone who has taken up a new sport or decided to shed some weight. It can also affect diabetics with NIDDM who are on antidiabetic medication.

Bernard was a big, jolly man who had always enjoyed his food and his whisky. He had been diabetic since he was 55, 10 years ago now. He had started on chlorpropamide (Diabinese) then. It seemed to suit him, so he was loath to change to another preparation when this was suggested, partly because of his age and partly because of his alcohol intake which was also increasing.

His family and friends were sad when Bernard began to deteriorate so rapidly. His memory lost its accuracy and his sense of humour its edge. He became careless, even sloppy, in areas of his life where he would have taken a pride before – his car, his garden, even his clothes.

'His whole personality has changed, and all the wrong way', his wife, Janet, explained. She was distressed. Bernard had become slack in monitoring his blood sugar – to tell the truth, he had never like this fiddly task. It was not until a routine biennial trip to the hospital, when Janet was with him, that the cause of his mental decline, a chronically low blood sugar level, was discovered.

The doctor told Bernard that he must stop taking the chlorpropamide, the longest-acting of the sulphonylurea medicines for diabetes.

The snag with a long-acting drug is that, if the dose is a little high, it takes so long for it to work through the system. Glibenclamide (Daonil) is much the same, and neither that nor chlorpropamide are suitable for older people. Among the safer drugs are gliclazide (Diamicron), glipizide (Glibenese) and tolbutamide (Rastinon). Hypoglycaemia is more likely to develop if there is any impairment of the liver (as turned out to be the case for Bernard as he had been quite a heavy drinker in his younger days) or the kidneys.

There are also some medicines that can tip the balance in favour of a hypoglycaemic state – for instance, aspirin, beta-blockers, sulphona-mides, and some antiarthritic and antigout drugs. You are more likely to use one of these as you get older. Hypoglycaemia in this age group may have effects on physical health. It puts a strain on the whole body and, if you have a heart or artery problem, it may make matters worse and cause chest pain, dizziness or a fit. These symptoms will probably subside when the blood sugar returns to normal.

Chronic hypoglycaemia is most frequently experienced by older NIDDM diabetics, but younger people may get it too. The symptoms can be fatigue, loss of muscle power and poor concentration. Check yourself out if you are under 40, diabetic and these symptoms have begun to bother you.

What to do Unlike acute hypoglycaemia, chronic hypoglycaemia isn't cured by a simple dose of sugar. It calls for a long, hard look at your lifestyle – what you eat and drink, how much exercise you take and what kind, the regularity of your day-to-day activities and what stresses there are in your life.

Prophylaxis

This means avoiding hypos or their ill-effects.
To do this:

- carry a card and/or wear a bracelet which says that you are a diabetic on insulin or whatever medication you are on
- make sure those you live and work with know the signs of a hypo and the emergency treatment for it
- take meticulously regular meals
- carry a pack of dextrose tablets in your pocket or bag
- check with your doctor about driving

- avoid high-risk sports, but you can have plenty of fun without hang-gliding, scuba diving or bungie-jumping.

9
Long-term Complications

As we saw in the last chapter, the complications of diabetes fall into two main groups. There are those such as ketoacidosis and hypoglycaemia that are direct, immediate reflections of the level of glucose in your blood, and a larger, more wide-ranging group. The latter are the long-term effects of the diabetic process. They require years to develop, although in NIDDM you may have been unaware of the shortfall of insulin for as long as seven years before the diagnosis was made and so they may have begun to occur. This contrasts with the situation in IDDM, which comes on so dramatically and unmistakably that there will be none of these problems for some years after you first learned that you were diabetic.

The long-term complications are essentially to do with the effects the disturbed sugar and fat metabolism have on the blood vessels. They are of two types:

- macrovascular, which means that they involve the big arteries
- microvascular, which means that they involve the small blood vessels, which nourish the various organs and systems of the body.

Macrovascular disorders

Atherosclerosis (the silting up of the arteries with fatty deposits) occurs in all of us as we get older, but it tends to start sooner in people with diabetes of either type. If the main channels for the blood are partly blocked – imagine city streets with badly parked vehicles on each side – the flow of vital supplies may be seriously impaired. The most important areas affected by this are:

- the brain, causing transient ischaemic attacks (TIAs) and, at the worst, a stroke
- the heart, causing disturbances to its action and even a heart attack
- the limbs, especially the legs and feet, causing pain.

TIAs
These are little warnings, that although harmless in themselves, mean you need to take action to improve the blood supply to your brain.

Shelagh was 67, an NIDDM sufferer whose treatment had consisted of diet and and tolbutamide during the seven years since the illness was discovered.

It was when she went to her granddaughter's wedding on a crisp October day that she had a 'funny turn'. The young couple had chosen a long wedding day, packed with events – the Church service in the morning, a reception and lunch filling half the afternoon – and an evening party when the cake would be cut, followed by a disco. Shelagh intended to miss the last item, but wanted to be there for the cutting of the cake and all the good wishes.

Champagne and sophisticated nibbles were on hand all day, but it was tiring, with a lot of standing. Shelagh was looking round for somewhere to sit down for a little while when a feeling of dizziness swept over her, she became unsteady on her feet and had to clutch at the wall. The oddest part was that she suddenly began to see double. The whole, strange experience only lasted a few minutes, then she was back to normal. Her doctor gave her a thorough check-up over the next day, including taking her blood pressure, checking her reflexes, giving her an electrocardiogram (ECG, which checks the functioning of the heart) and a blood test.

He told Shelagh that her blood sugar was out of kilter, probably made worse by the rich foods at the wedding, and that her blood pressure was definitely too high. He explained that she had suffered a TIA, Nature's signal to take steps to avoid the risk of a stroke.

Basil's warning was an abnormal ECG, done as a routine part of his firm's annual medical for executives. They told him he was in line for a coronary if he didn't take care. Basil was 55 and had added two additional risk factors to his diabetes: smoking cheroots and drinking alcohol regularly.

Both Basil and Shelagh were overweight, and, in his case, it was more serious as the surplus was high on his abdomen. Here it is far more likely to cause trouble than where Shelagh's excess fat was, under the skin round her hips and thighs.

For both Shelagh and Basil, there were now clear guidelines for them to follow if they were to stave off the major dangers facing them:

- smoking was right out
- alcohol, because of its ill-effects on diabetes, weight problems and blood pressure, was to be reduced significantly
- losing weight was a must – Basil and Shelagh each needed to shed about 6 kg (1 stone), not by crash dieting but by consistently controlling what they ate. Shelagh was set a 1,000-calorie intake, Basil, 1,200, with 50 per cent of it to be in high fibre, unrefined carbohydrates, very little to be in saturated fat, and around 10 to 15 per cent of it protein (see page 47).

Beneficial effects of losing at least 10 per cent of your original weight are:

- better blood sugar control
- increased sensitivity to insulin
- a much-reduced risk of advancing atherosclerosis.

In spite of having smaller meals more often and more evenly throughout the day, Basil felt miserably deprived, particularly as he had given up smoking and nearly all alcohol. So his doctor suggested that he might like to try metformin instead of the glipizide he was then taking. Metformin is an antidiabetic medicine that differs chemically from others (see page 52). It doesn't suit everyone, but it helps people lose weight. Some people lose all appetite while they are on it and a few have diarrhoea. Basil had neither side-effect, and brought his body mass index down to an acceptable 27 (see page 117).

Shelagh was not as successful and her doctor finally decided to start her on insulin.

High blood pressure

High blood pressure, or hypertension, is not a direct complication of diabetes, but it is frequently associated with it. There may a genetic link with NIDDM. Hypertension greatly increases the dangers of athero-sclerosis and also puts a strain on the kidneys. The latter are already at risk of damage from the excess sugar passing through them.

Blood pressure, including high blood pressure, is expressed in millimetres of mercury, like atmospheric pressure. It comprises two numbers. The first denotes the pressure in the arteries when the heart is in mid-pump, or systole, actually driving the blood round. The second, lower figure represents the pressure during diastole, that is, when the heart is relaxing between beats. A normal pressure would be, say, 135/ 80. The World Health Organization criteria for blood pressure are:

	Systolic	Diastolic
Normal	*less than 140*	*less than 90*
Borderline	*140 to 160*	*90 to 95*
High	*more than 160*	*more than 95*

Hypertension is more prevalent among diabetics with IDDM than the general population, especially if they are over 50. It is even commoner in those with NIDDM, affecting nearly half of them. Women are more likely to be sufferers than men, and dark-skinned people of either sex likelier still, whether they are Asian, African or Caribbean. One third of people in Oxford, newly diagnosed as being diabetic, were found to have blood pressures above the safety limit of 160/95 already. Their GPs did not know. The snag is that, although it may be having undesirable long-term effects, someone with a rising blood pressure may feel perfectly well for years.

> Felicity who, truth to tell, was something of a hypochondriac, was one of those rare people to detect and report to her doctor two mild, occasional symptoms of hypertension. She had headaches now and again and was passing water more often than she used to. This latter, of course, is also a symptom of diabetes, which makes it difficult for a diabetic to spot hypertension. The doctor found that Felicity had a high blood glucose level and her blood pressure was 168/97.
>
> Felicity was 50 at this point and worked in a library – a job she found to be very stressful. For her 'bad heads' she swallowed generous amounts of an over-the-counter painkiller of the non-steroidal anti-inflammatory drug (NSAID) type. By chance, it was one of a handful of drugs that tends to push blood pressure up. When she substituted paracetamol, her blood pressure went down to the borderline OK level.

Other medicines that may raise your blood pressure include the Pill when it contains oestrogen, steroids, such as prednisolone, some asthma inhalers and some indigestion mixtures.

High blood pressure makes all macrovascular problems worse, as well as increasing the risk to kidneys and eyes, so it must be brought under control. To do this:

- if you are overweight, aim to get your body mass index down to 27 or less (see page 117)
- drastically reduce your intake of alcohol or give it up altogether
- do not add salt to your food
- find some technique – whether it is yoga or watching television – that helps you to relax
- do not smoke
- take regular, mild exercise, such as golf or walking rather than squash.
- take the medicines prescribed, but check they are OK with diabetes.

The standard initial treatment for hypertension is to take thiazide water tablets and beta-blockers. These are fine if you don't have diabetes, but both are best avoided if you do. Other medicines that lower the blood pressure are nifedipine (Adalat), verapamil (Securan), doxazosin (Cardura) and captopril (Capoten). They each achieve the desired effect in different ways, but do not interfere with the control of your blood sugar nor your erections, if you are a man, unlike the standard treatment. It is a balancing act for your diabetic specialist, selecting the drug to suit your individual situation, one that will control your blood pressure without having troublesome side-effects. There is a long-running discussion among diabetologists over the merits and demerits of each medicine.

Mubariz had been diabetic since he was 20. At this point he was 38. He worked very hard and very late in a nightclub and he had to carefully juggle his insulin and meals to control his blood glucose with such unsocial hours. He often felt exhausted and, finally, Josie persuaded him to see his GP for a check-up.

Mubariz learned that his blood pressure was up, at 170/90, and that there was a trace of protein in his water, indicating that strain was being put on his kidneys. The kidneys are particularly vulnerable to damage from hypertension if you are diabetic.

The aim was to get Mubariz' reading down to 130–140/80–85. This was achieved by Mubariz taking captopril plus continuing to monitor his blood sugar level carefully, aiming at a target of 8 mmol/1. He was not overweight, so there was no need for him to cut down his food. However, he is now on the look-out for a job with more civilized hours, even if it means a drop in income.

LONG-TERM COMPLICATIONS

Angela presented a different problem. She was 69 and had had diabetes for 14 years. Since Bernard had retired, she'd had to do a lot more cooking and she relaxed her own eating a little. She developed a late midde-age spread and her glucose level often passed the upper limit of 11 mmol/l, but so long as she felt well she didn't worry.

It was the chest pain that she felt when she was walking uphill or after Sunday dinner that sent her to the doctor. She told Angela that her blood pressure was far too high, at 200/110, and that she judged that the arteries had been narrowed by atherosclerosis. It was the stress on Angela's heart, working against pressure with a limited blood supply, that was causing this anginal pain.

Angela has glyceryltrinitate (GTN) tablets to ward off the angina, but her doctor is considering trying Angela on icarol, a newer anti-angina medicine that is suitable for diabetics and has no side-effects. To lower her blood pressure, Angela takes doxazosin. Originally she had tried verapamil, which is meant to help with both hypertension and angina, but it made her too constipated. Doxazosin has no such troublesome side-effects, and helps when there is an excess of fat in the blood, which seems likely in Angela's case.

Just as important as the medication are some sensible adjustments to Angela's lifestyle. She needs to apply a little restraint in her diet, aiming at a gradual, long-term reduction in weight, plus a daily walk to the park or the shops, say, if only to buy a paper. Gentle exercise improves the blood supply to the heart and muscles, but it is not wise to exert yourself just after a meal.

Pain in the legs

The main arteries to the limbs may also be silted up which is known as peripheral vascular disease. A shortage of blood to the calf muscles makes them hurt when you try to make them work hard, for instance when going upstairs. This is the equivalent of angina, when the heart muscle is deprived, but the calves may also be painful in the night.

Diabetes is not the only cause of this problem. Smoking alone may be responsible in susceptible people, so if you have even a whisper of calf pain, you absolutely must not smoke. Keeping the amount of fat in your diet down is also important. Exercise, short of causing discomfort, is beneficial, as is taking extra care to control your glucose level. In some cases, surgical techniques can greatly improve the blood flow, but you still have to apply these general measures.

Painful calf muscles naturally make you limp at times, which has the impressive name of intermittent claudication. Obviously, if the arteries in your legs are not healthy, the blood supply to your feet is poor and they are at risk (see Chapter 10).

Microvascular disorders

It is only in diabetes that the smallest – micro – blood vessels, the capillaries, are subject to damage and blocking all over the body. There are probably other factors involved as well as the excess sugar going through them, but strictly controlling the amount of sugar in the blood does help to prevent this damage occurring.

Both the IDDM and the NIDDM sufferers are affected, but, either way, only after the diabetic process has been underway for several years. The parts at risk as a result of microvascular damage are:

- the eyes
- the kidneys
- the nerves
- the feet.

The first three parts are discussed below, while the feet are covered in the next chapter.

Eye problems

Blurred vision It is not unusual to get a slight blurring of vision when you first develop diabetes and your treatment regimen is not yet established. This is a nuisance, but not a threat. If you have too much sugar in your blood, this also seeps into the fluid inside your eye, through which you see. It is like looking through syrup. When the sugar level in your blood comes under control, the eye fluid corrects itself in due time. However, if the change is too sudden, it makes your sight temporarily worse. Steady adjustment and patience are the ideal approach.

This problem is unimportant and passes, but there can be serious risks to your eyesight if you suffer microvascular disease. It is a sobering thought that diabetes is the commonest cause of blindness among adults of working age in Britain and other First-World countries. The plus side is that it is possible to prevent it. Adhering strictly to the rules for healthy diabetic living will mean successfully averting eye disorders in 70 per cent of cases, so it is under your control.

Even if your eyes have suffered some damage, if you take your lifestyle in hand at an early stage, you can put the clock back. Finally, if the damage is more severe, there is effective, almost magical treatment available using lasers.

You must have regular eye checks as soon as you know you have diabetes, otherwise you may be unaware that you need treatment. Like so much in diabetes, you may have no symptoms to alert you that trouble is brewing, but a doctor looking into the back of your eye will pick up the smallest signs. Then the problem can be treated before it gets worse.

Ben didn't like doctors – he thought of them as being only one step up from tax inspectors. He resented his diabetes, too. It had come upon him when he was 15, after his mother had been killed on a zebra crossing.

At the age of 25, he was busy building up a reputation for making scientific documentaries when he was suddenly panicked by the thought that if his diabetes affected his sight, his career, in this most visual of industries, would be finished.

First, he went to an optician, who told him that he didn't need glasses, but he wasn't satisfied. Nor did he feel reassured when his GP offered to 'take a squint' through his ophthalmoscope. He insisted on consulting an eye surgeon and his persistence paid off.

The opthalmic registrar detected some minute, dark red spots on Ben's retina, the lining at the back of his eye, which is fundamental to the ability to see. The spots were tiny bulges in the delicate capillaries, which were due to small blockages.

These full-stop-sized bulges, or aneurysms, are the very earliest sign of diabetic damage to the eyes, or diabetic retinopathy. At this stage, all that Ben needed was to review the management of his diabetes, with a view to keeping his blood glucose between 3.9 and 6.7 mmol/l before meals and no more than 10 mmol/l after. He had two injections of insulin daily, but was prepared to have more if necessary.

All this was five years ago and now his work regularly appears on television. His retinopathy has not advanced and his sight is unimpaired.

In fact, it is still soon enough to prevent the development of serious retinopathy if your eyes show little leaks of blood or plasma as well as tiny aneurysms when they are examined. Even if this is the case, you will probably have been unaware of any interference with your sight.

The longer you keep up strict control of your diabetes, the safer your eyes are, year by year. Regular examinations are also an essential part of the routine.

Pre-proliferative or pre-malignant retinopathy is a stage worse. The term 'malignant' here has nothing to do with cancer, but merely means that it is dangerous. The 'pre' means it is not *yet* dangerous, but watch out. While an interested family doctor may monitor the health of your eyes effectively up to this stage, if this condition is found it is essential to see a specialist. At this point, the macula – the most sensitive part of the retina – may be swollen and you find you cannot focus properly. Maculopathy, as it is called, crops up most frequently in those with NIDDM. If it occurs, it isn't an emergency, but you must get first-class advice and treatment quickly.

Even if the macula isn't affected, the retina may show relatively big haemorrhages and a lot of plasma oozing into the special fluid of your eye. If you have slipped into the phase of pre-proliferative retinal trouble, taking firm control of your diabetes still gives you a better than 50:50 chance of halting a downhill progression. The judicious use of laser treatment is dramatically helpful here, too.

Proliferative retinopathy, which means a serious threat to your sight, is an attempt by the eye to heal the damaged retina by producing new blood vessels and fibrous scar tissue. This causes real problems as the new vessels easily bleed into the eye fluid and the fibrous tissue tends to drag parts of the retina from its attachments.

Urgent ophthalmic treatment is mandatory because without it there would be a high risk of blindness following within a few years. Laser treatment seals off leaking vessels, but cannot always work if there is too much fibrous tissue in the way, so it is important to catch it as early as possible.

Gareth was one of the unlucky ones. He was in his sixties, a drinking, smoking, eating, jokey extrovert. He liked to believe that because he didn't need insulin, he had only a 'mild' form of diabetes. He didn't take much account of his blood pressure, either. It wasn't seriously up, but his doctor had told him it was higher than was healthy.

Gareth's sight wasn't wonderful, but caused him no real inconvenience until, out of the blue, a black film blotted out his vision on the left and some black floaters got in the way on the right. Both conditions were the effects of bleeding into the eye fluid, an emergency situation. Gareth lost most of his sight.

Sometimes surgery – either vitrectomy (removal of the affected eye fluid) or membrane stripping – can restore some vision, even to an eye that was blind. At the worst, there is other help available and you are not alone in your predicament. There are 1.75 million people in the UK with significantly impaired sight (see page 91).

Glaucoma This is an increase of pressure inside the eye, which affects diabetics more often than other people. Indications are seeing a halo effect around lights, having blurred vision and eye-ache. This may escalate until you have a tense, red, painful eye.

If you even *suspect* glaucoma, go to your doctor straight away. A tonometer will measure the eye pressure simply. Glaucoma endangers your sight, but there is effective treatment to hand.

Cataracts These, too, are rather more frequent among diabetics than others, and are likely to develop earlier if blood sugar control is lax.

Part of your field of vision will be blurred if you have a cataract and an additional snag for diabetics is that the doctor cannot get a good view of the retina because the lens of the eye becomes misty. This means, though, that your cataract operation is likely to be undertaken sooner than most, which is a bonus. There is no reason, stemming from the diabetes, for you not to have a new lens inserted if this is what is required.

If you are diabetic, you need to take particular care of your eyesight – care in terms of controlling your diabetes, having regular eye examinations, even if you have no symptoms, and avoiding extra risk factors, which are smoking, poorly controlled high blood pressure, using the Pill, drinking alcohol in excess and neglecting signs of kidney trouble.

Kidney problems

Your urinary system comprises the kidneys, which collect waste products from the blood, the bladder, used for temporary storage, and the tubes connecting up the whole system. Problems in one part affect the others, which is why cystitis is an important infection.

Cystitis This is a commonplace infection of the bladder, affecting women more often than men as it is easier for bacteria to travel up the comparatively short, straight tube to the bladder in the female than in the male.

Because, as a diabetic, you are prone to have a little sugar in your water, the unwanted bacteria are more likely to flourish than otherwise.

You know you have cystitis if you have aching pain low in your abdomen and a burning sensation when you pass water. Your urine may be tinged with blood, look cloudy or smell bad.

Antibiotics provide a quick, effective cure most of the time, but if you are unlucky enough to fall into a cycle of cystitis, antibiotic, cystitis, you can break the pattern by taking long-term, low-dose medication. You must, anyway, be meticulous about hygiene in the crucial area, not using harsh soaps, but plenty of plain, warm water. Always wash after a bowel movement and wipe from the front towards the back to avoid taking bacteria from the stools to the urethra.

Kidney infections Sometimes, an infection can extend up into the kidney. This is highly undesirable with diabetes, when the kidneys are already under strain. Kidney infections make you feel thoroughly ill, with a fever and pain in the back. As well as the antibiotic to deal with the bacteria, you may need extra insulin until the illness subsides.

Infections are troublesome in the short term, but what matters more is the specific disorder of diabetic nephropathy. Damage to the tiniest blood vessels – microvascular disease – interferes with the working of the kidneys. Fortunately, they have a vast reserve. For example, many people have only one kidney and are perfectly well. Even if the capillary vessels are being affected, it will be many years, if ever, before the system loses its efficiency.

It is those who were under 30 when their diabetes developed who run the greatest risk as they have a great stretch of life ahead of them during which kidney damage can develop. As many as 30 to 40 per cent of those with IDDM, compared with 20 per cent of those with NIDDM may reach the stage of nephropathy. Also, as with high blood pressure, black-or brown-skinned people are especially vulnerable.

If no action is taken in the early stages, the results can be serious. As with all microvascular problems, carefully controlling blood glucose levels right from the very beginning is a protection. Equally vital is having regular checks, at least once a year, however well you feel. Checking your eyes and kidneys is most important when you have been diabetic for five years or more, which is time enough for early warning signs to be detectable by the tests.

Microproteinuria This is the leakage into the urine of miniscule amounts of protein, including albumen. This is a valuable advance warning of kidney stress. At first, it only shows up after exercise, but later on it is continuous and the amount of protein present is large enough to show up on a basic dipstick urine test.

Martina was a whizzkid at work and, perhaps because of her name, a keen tennis player. She had been diabetic since the age of ten, and now, at 27, she lived a full, active life. She was determined not to miss any opportunity and knew that she had to keep the diabetes licked to achieve her ambitions.

A trace of protein showed up in her urine in one of her regular check-ups during a tournament. It was a nuisance, but at least she was forewarned. From then on, she had more frequent tests and, as the microproteinuria gradually developed, she decided to deal with it.

Martina had read about the DCCT research in America (see page 10). This had shown conclusively that keeping tight control of blood glucose levels greatly reduced the risk of eye, nerve and kidney problems. Martina set about keeping her blood sugar really low. The down side of this was that she didn't always get enough warning of an impending hypo, and then she experienced a frighteningly severe attack. If she had been living alone, this could have been dangerous. As it was, she was advised never to let her glucose reading fall below 4 mmol/l, which seemed the lowest safe level for her.

She had also decided to cut down her protein intake to 65 g ($2\frac{1}{2}$ oz) daily, to reduce the workload for her kidneys. However, new research in the USA shows that such a restriction isn't necessary until a later stage in the disorder. If you cut your protein down, make sure that what you *do* have is genuinely first-class – milk, eggs, meat and liver.

The results of Martina's efforts have been rewarding. The degree of protein leakage in her urine has increased very little over the last few years. Incidentally, her eyes have benefited from the tight glucose control. Nearly everyone whose kidneys have been affected by a microvascular problem also have the beginnings of background retinopathy. Martina has no symptoms in either her eyes or her urinary system – for all practical purposes, they are working normally. The key is regular checks, even when there seems to be no reason to bother.

Not many of us are as obsessionally careful as Martina. We may either have remained unaware of the silent progress of kidney damage or have been unable to apply such rigid control. Also, such control is too risky in the case of young children or the elderly who are less likely to be aware of the first subtle indications of a hypo and to act on them quickly and efficiently.

High blood pressure It may be getting on for 20 years since you were diagnosed as being diabetic before you notice any physical symptoms, and you have the chance, during most of that time, to slow down any kidney damage by healthy diabetic living. An increase in blood pressure can be either the cause or the result of kidney strain. Unless you are definitely old, in which case you have proved yourself to be tough, if the lower figure in your blood pressure reaches 95, it is time to take action to reduce it (see page 88).

Other symptoms The symptoms of a kidney in trouble don't point directly to their source. For example, you may find that your blood sugar, which had been reasonably steady, is now all over the place. Often you have to reduce your insulin. Other indications are:

- lack of energy, mental and physical
- headaches
- nausea
- itchy skin.

These all show that waste products aren't being cleared efficiently through the kidneys. Sometimes the main problem is that they are letting too much protein through. In this case, you may get a build-up of fluid, which shows up as swelling in your face and ankles and may also make you short of breath.

Norman managed moderately well despite some kidney impairment for several years. Then he started feeling out-of-sorts most of the time and tired and miserable with it. At 47 he couldn't afford, and didn't want, to give up his job at the pharmacy. He asked if he should go on haemodialysis, which is when you are linked up to a machine that 'cleans' your blood. This method isn't ideal for diabetics as the anticlotting chemical in the dialysis fluid may increase the risk of bleeding in the retina.

Norman's specialist advised him to try Continuous Ambulatory Peritoneal Dialysis (CAPD). With this method, your system is cleansed four times a day via a tube fixed into your abdomen, and the beauty of it is that you can go about your normal life throughout the procedure. Children and older people cope with this form of dialysis well and it suits diabetics, too. Norman has had this treatment for two years now, but is on the list for a transplant. His diabetes will not disadvantage him when the transplant takes place.

Nerve problems

You have two separate systems of nerves:

- somatic
- autonomic.

The somatic system is the one you are aware of, bringing you information about touch, warmth or pain from all over the body and enabling you to send messages out to your muscles so that you can move around at will.

The autonomic system works automatically and you have no control over it. It regulates your heartbeat and blood pressure, your digestion and perspiration. For men, it must be in working order to effect an erection.

Like the eyes and the kidneys, the nerves are susceptible to damage if there is too much sugar in the blood and a general shortage of oxygen and nourishment because the smallest blood vessels are getting blocked up.

Symptoms of somatic nerve system damage

SENSATION The information arrangements may be upset – the commonest nerve problem in diabetes. The hands and feet, and sometimes the front of the abdomen, are the parts that are most often affected. These areas may, very gradually, go numb – so-called glove and stocking anaesthesia. Apart from feeling weird when you walk, there is a danger of cutting or knocking yourself without realizing that you have done so. This means taking extra care, especially of your feet.

Less often, instead of a loss of feeling, the nerves may play up in the *opposite* way, so that you may be extra-sensitive to the slightest touch or have pins and needles. Some people suffer distressing pain in the parts affected.

It is not much consolation to know that these various unpleasant sensations are due the nerves struggling to 'come to life'. The better news is that the condition is intermittent, and usually clears up altogether within a few months.

Meanwhile, you need medication to relieve any pain and there is a wide choice:

- the usual painkillers, such as paracetamol and ibuprofen and, on prescription, co-proxamol
- the antidepressent amitriptyline, in a small dose – for its effect on the nervous tissue, not your mood
- fluphenazine, a tranquillizer, for similar reasons
- carbamazepine or phenytoin, antiepileptic drugs, similarly
- transcutaneous electrical nerve stimulation (TENS), which works wonderfully well for pain, but not for everyone.

MOVEMENT If the nerves that are under stress are those supplying your muscles, the effect will be weakness, for instance of finger or foot movements, and, occasionally, in a big muscle in the thigh.

These somatic nerve difficulties nearly always affect more than one part and so they are called poly-neuropathies – 'poly' meaning 'many'. There is no tailor-made treatment for dealing with them, but good control of your diabetes helps, together with whatever measures ease the particular problems. What is vital is preventative care, that is, having frequent examinations and taking great care of your feet (see the next chapter).

Symptoms of autonomic nerve system damage You will not experience all of the following, but it is useful to know what to look for and to be able to recognize the cause if you do have any of them:

- the ability to exercise is limited because your heart rate isn't fully responsive to the needs of the moment
- feeling dizzy when you stand up quickly because your blood pressure doesn't react as quickly as usual to your change of position
- heartburn, poor appetite and/or bloating because the system is

regulating the digestive system less efficiently (metoclopramide may be a helpful medicine in this case, and it is wiser *not* to go for a high-fibre diet, with loads of roughage, vegetables and fruit.)

- bowel disturbance (60 per cent of diabetics are liable to be constipated, requiring exercise and mild laxatives; a few have diarrhoea instead, mainly at night)
- embarrassing sweating of your face and head, especially after even a small meal, which is linked with too little perspiration everywhere else, so that you cannot tolerate excessive heat
- problems with achieving an erection (see page 59).

Any of these may be a nuisance, but, as with the symptoms of somatic nerve damage, there is no neat cure. Again, general measures are beneficial and don't omit to look after your feet. See how in the next chapter.

10

Your Feet

Babies are fascinated by their feet, waving them around and trying to catch them. You may not regard your feet as particularly interesting or particularly romantic now, but they are essential for every part of your daily activities and they transport you to the shops, from bedroom to kitchen, from here to there. They deserve credit for what they do for you – and consideration.

Especially, they need due consideration when you are diabetic. They run 25 times the risk of other people's feet of one day requiring amputation. Diabetes creates a two-pronged attack on them:

- damage to the nerve supply
- damage to the blood supply

Either complication makes them vulnerable to infection. Fortunately, there is plenty you can do to prevent your feet falling victim to anything too nasty. The proof of this is that many diabetics who have had the condition for 30 or 40 years have feet that give them no trouble at all. You can avoid any major problems by nipping minor ones in the bud.

Ideally, you should monitor the well-being of your feet from the day you know you are diabetic. If you did not do this then, why not start today?

The routine physical examination at the clinic or surgery includes a detailed look at your feet, but the real responsibility lies with you. Make it a habit to give them a once-over every day. You do it with your face and hair, so why not your feet, too? This kind of attention obviously becomes increasingly advisable as you get older, when wear-and-tear effects may begin to show, but it matters for those under 30, too. Sport, for example, can give your feet a hard time – they must be 100 per cent fit for that.

Factors that increase the risks

These are as follows:
- if you are over 40
- if you smoke

- if you have had diabetes for ten years or more
- if you have slightly less feeling in your feet than in other parts
- if you have any existing conditions, such as a bunion, hammer toe or claw toe
- if you have any injury, however trivial.

Luckily there are plenty of signs and symptoms to alert you to possible, impending problems – in time to do something about them.

What to look out for

- *Indications of nerve damage*:
  - warm, pink feet, later becoming cold
  - dry skin with a tendency to cracks and fissures, because the nerves that cause the skin to sweat aren't working
  - the gradual dulling of sensation (this is common but dangerous, as you may not feel it if there is a flint or a nail sticking up in your shoe, even if it injures your foot, and you may be unaware if an ill-fitting shoe is rubbing or if you have a deep crack in the skin that becomes infected
  - calluses or patches of thickened skin, caused by pressure, which are often found under the foot or at the tips of your toes
  - painless ulcers, usually developing as a result of breakdown of tissue under a callus spreading and becoming infected. (Ulcers can, especially if injured, develop into gangrene, so these are a very important sign)
  - swelling of the foot
  - extra-sensitivity of the skin next to an area of numbness where even the lightest touch may feel peculiarly unpleasant
  - instead of dulled sensation, you may get periods of intense burning, stabbing or deep, bone-aching pain
  - weakness in the muscles so that your foot may tend to sag; your hands may feel weak as well
  - unsteadiness when you are walking, because of damage to the nerves that tell you where your limbs and feet are
  - changes in your toes, so that, over the years, gradually they don't lie flat, but curve downwards.
- *Indications of poor blood supply*:
  - cold feet

- when the skin is a pale colour when you lift your feet, but they turn purple when they hang down
- pain or throbbing in your feet, especially at night, because not enough blood is getting to them (you can get some temporary relief for a few minutes by hanging your legs down over the side of the bed, because this allows blood from the veins to run back into the feet under the influence of gravity)
- limping because of pain in your feet and, sometimes, in your calf muscles (see page 90)
- the borders of your feet feel more uncomfortable than the middle.
- *Effects on the skin*:
  - it is either extra painful or oddly painless when you suffer injuries
  - very slow healing of any injury
  - dry, itchy, scaly skin
  - corns and hard patches
  - infections between the toes, round the nails and in cracks and ulcers, which may look red and inflamed without your feeling sore.

Any one of these warning signs should send you straight to your doctor or directly to the diabetic clinic for an MOT of your feet and advice on what action is necessary.

Jennifer had difficulty keeping a watch on her feet. Arthritis in her hips and knees prevented her from getting close enough to have a good look. Added to that, she was developing cataracts, which slightly blurred her field of vision. She could feel with her fingers that there was a hard place under the ball of her left big toe, but even with a mirror she could not get a good view of it. As she said, she felt she had been divorced from her feet. There was no way that she could see them properly, and, even with long-handled scissors, she could not feel confident about cutting her nails.

Although Jennifer was only 72, she had been a widow for 6 years, and her daughter, now in her forties, lived miles away with a family of her own. Jennifer did not know her neighbours well enough to ask them to take over the monitoring of her feet.

The answer for Jennifer was to see the practice nurse, with expert back-up from a chiropodist. The latter was available to Jennifer on the NHS as she was a pensioner and diabetic.

What your doctor can do for your feet

Of course, your doctor will keep a check on your diabetes, your blood pressure and your general health before focusing on your feet. As well as looking for all the warning signs mentioned so far, your doctor will also make a special examination:

- feeling for the pulse in the arteries in the groin, behind the knee and on the top of the foot
- listening for a sound called a bruit, when the blood has a restricted passageway over your main thigh artery
- testing your reflexes – that your knee and ankle jerks when tapped
- testing for sensation in your feet and lower legs by:
  - moving your big toe while your eyes are shut to see if you can sense its position by means of nerve information alone
  - brushing your skin with a wisp of cotton wool, to test that you feel a light touch
  - touching you with the point or the head of a pin, to see that you can feel pain
  - touching you with a cold and a warm object, to check that you can sense temperature
  - holding a tuning fork against your ankle bones to see if you sense the vibration
  - trying your muscles out to detect any weakness
  - pressing your skin with a finger and seeing how long it takes for the blood to come back into the white fingermark created by the pressure.

There is also a range of special tests to detect any artery problems.

The professional people you may come across

The following experts may be needed at any point depending on your circumstances:

- your own doctor
- specialist physician
- orthopaedic surgeon
- vascular surgeon
- chiropodist
- shoe-fitting expert
- nurse.

104

How to deal with injuries

For anything other than a minor, uninfected injury (see page 106 for how to handle these) you will require help from a specialist in diabetic foot care. You might need: treatment with medication to relieve any pain; shoes designed for your feet to redistribute the pressure alongside resting them and applying a walking plaster; antibiotics, including some for deeply situated bacteria; antifungal treatment; operations on your leg arteries, including bypassing blocked sections or repairing a blood vessel; dealing with callouses and corns by chiropody; orthopaedic operations for hammer toes or other problems with the bones, or if the worst comes to the worst and gangrene sets in, the affected part may have to be removed.

Common-sense rules for keeping your feet happy and healthy

Take heart! None of these symptoms and things that could go wrong with your feet need apply to you. Look after your feet and they should be fine. Here are some guidelines to follow.

- Have a annual medical examination.
- Give your feet a daily once-over.
- Daily, wash them with warm water and a very little baby soap. Don't soak them.
- Dry your feet gently, including between the toes. Lightly dust them with talc to make sure they are really dry.
- Wear clean socks, stockings or tights every day.
- Discard any socks or other footwear that cramp your toes.
- Cut your nails straight across and not too short. If you have any difficulty doing this, get someone else to do it (your partner, a good friend, chiropodist or nurse).
- Massage moisturizing cream sparingly into your feet if the skin is dry.
- If your feet get cold and wet, dry them, put on dry socks and shoes, but don't then toast them by a heater.
- Avoid very hot baths, hotwater bottles and electric blankets, except to take the chill off the bedclothes before you go to bed.
- For corns and hard patches, don't use corn plasters or solvents and don't try and cut them off. Get professional care.

- For small cuts or scratches, clean the area with a very little amount of soap and some water, then dry and put on a dry dressing.
- For a blister, treat it as though it were a small cut. *Don't* pop it!
- Don't use a plaster over a sore or injured place, although you can use it at the side to anchor a dry dressing.
- Don't use strong antiseptics – they are too harsh.
- Take real care when buying your shoes. Get expert help and make sure that your shoes are deep enough and wide enough and are comfortable without the need for any 'breaking in'. Avoid high heels and go for soft leather or canvas uppers. Lace-ups give the best support, while slip-ons and slippers give none.
- Don't walk around indoors without anything on your feet.

Some general precautions

As nicotine has such a devastating effect on the arteries, it is vital that you don't smoke. If necessary, use nicotine patches to break your habit.

For the nerves as well as the blood vessels, aim to keep your blood glucose between 4 and 8 mmol/l, which means you hardly ever have a positive urine test. If you have NIDDM and you are middle-aged, check with your doctor whether you should have a higher limit for your glucose.

Everything that is good for your general well-being will be good for your feet. Keep yourself fit and healthy from head to toe.

11

Moods and Feelings

Your mind and your body together make up the essential you. There is a continuous interplay between these two aspects, each affecting the other. It is an everyday experience that if, for instance, you have toothache, you can't concentrate, you can't relax and, if it is bad enough, you feel miserable. Equally, when you are excited or afraid, you can feel your heart beating faster. This cause and effect relationship exists in diabetes, too – your feelings influence the illness and vice versa.

Before you develop diabetes

It is a statistical fact that diabetics are likely to have had more upsetting experiences and conflicts than other people during the three years before the disorder comes out. Bereavements, losing your job, moving house, especially to a new locality, someone you love being ill, financial stringency, divorce, failing an exam – all these count.

Personality and stress

Back in the 1930s, Dr Flanders Dunbar had a theory that there was a particular personality that went with diabetes: 'weak, irritable, hypochondriacal and changeable'. It has been shown since Dunbar's day, however, that there is absolutely no validity in his notion. What he saw was the run-up stage experienced with any illness, that time when you don't feel right but can't tell what is wrong. You can develop diabetes *whatever* your personality, but different types have different ways of coping.

In general, the thoughtful introverts are the most meticulous in managing their health, but are likely to brood over possible snags and difficulties. The bubbly, sociable extroverts, by contrast, have a more carefree attitude, but may chafe at keeping to a diabetic routine.

In the seventeenth century, doctors believed that a long-continued state of unhappiness could lead to diabetes, while, in the nineteenth century, Henry Maudsley of the famous psychiatric hospital in London considered that 'violent passions' triggered the disorder. In the same

Victorian period, Dr R. T. Williamson blamed 'loss of money or employment' for 10 per cent of cases, and 'overwork, especially looking after a sick relative' for another 8 per cent. In our own century, American doctors Stein and Charles showed that there was an excess of family conflict in the background of many future diabetics.

All these views were sometimes right, but the acute emotional upset put forward by Maudsley is a more potent risk than mild, long-term worry. Heartbreak, fear and anger are the worst emotions for your health.

Alfred was burgled. What made him furious was that the intruders struck when he was in hospital having a prostate operation. He came home for rest and quiet to find his little bungalow in chaos and the television and microwave gone. As a widower, Alfred depended on these two items more than most. His diabetes started to develop during the next few weeks.

Malcolm, aged ten, also developed diabetes after experiencing a shock, in his case that of finding his father dead (see page 4).

The body's response to stress is the same as its response to danger. It increases the amounts of glucose and fat in the blood. This ensures a plentiful supply of fuel for the muscles for fighting or running away. The response is the same even when the stress is purely mental and the muscles won't be burning up the extra glucose. This means a prolonged demand for extra insulin, which may be too much of a strain. The worst time for a stressful event to occur as far as your body is concerned is just after a big meal.

Emotional disturbances are also damaging when you have established diabetes. The blood sugar level goes up and your normal routine for controlling it fails. If you are living through a period of psychological turmoil, and especially if you are diabetic or at risk, it is worth seeking out help to alleviate the situation (see page 33).

When you hear that you are diabetic

It is bound to have an impact, realizing that you have an illness that will be with you forever and involves a shake-up of your whole way of life. Of course, you will adapt and get your balance back, but, meanwhile, you will go through an emotional journey that can be rather like that of a bereavement.

First of all, it doesn't seem real – you can't take in the diagnosis and all it implies. Then you may feel angry – why *me*? You may blame yourself, your parents, fate or the illness itself. Your indignation can spill over on to doctors, nurses, your nearest and dearest. Later, a mood of depression may sweep over you. You may feel less of a person, as though you have been punished, and insecure about the future.

This distressing process of coming to terms with your diabetes is usually short-lived, and your natural coping abilities take over. However, if you were already vulnerable and the diabetes is the final straw, adapting to it may be more difficult.

- *Emotional reactions* These may include feeling threatened and under pressure. You may be unable to settle, and tearful and worn out from the moment you wake up. Everything may look black.
- *Your physical state* Your appetite may dwindle, you may be unable to sleep and lie drenched in sweat, and you may get pins and needles round your mouth and in your fingers – these are symptoms of anxiety. Headaches, stomachaches and chest pain fall into this same category.

In this state you cannot feel normally towards other people who are not diabetic. You may shrink from contact with them or, conversely, crave their company all the time, to reassure yourself that you are human, too. You may go to extremes with sex also – losing all interest or wanting it unusually often.

Leslie was the type to bottle up his feelings. He seemed to take the news with equanimity, that his weakness and weight loss were down to diabetes. While his pals and his parents admired the way he was taking it in his stride, Leslie's inner emotions were in a turmoil of anger and despair. Although the professionals explained the facts, as he didn't communicate how he felt, they did not give him the support and reassurance he needed. He dropped out of his normal social activities, dumped his girlfriend and spent hours in his room, ostensibly studying. This might have gone on indefinitely if his grandmother hadn't come to stay. She was 80, and she had always had a soft spot for Leslie. She helped him to unlock his fear and unhappiness. This marked the beginning of his recovery process.

If you are having trouble adapting to the new, difficult concept of being a diabetic, don't suffer in silence. Talking about it takes out the sting. Tell your relatives and friends – you need their tender loving care. Tell your doctor, the diabetes nurse and any other professional involved. You need to have regular discussions with people who know about diabetes. Even if you have a bad dose of adaptation blues, if you share the burden, it will lift inside a couple of months. Yoga or formal relaxation classes can help if you are particularly tense.

Psychological problems that may affect diabetics

Taken over a lifetime, diabetics suffer no more psychological problems than do members of the general population, but that amounts to between 30 and 40 per cent. It can be a puzzle to distinguish symptoms due to diabetes from those due to depression or anxiety, which require different treatment.

Depression

This is the commonest upset, and usually includes some anxiety. It can affect any age and either sex, but women are twice as susceptible as men and overweight women are more vulnerable than others.

Often the person's partner is the first to realize that something is wrong. Early signs are a general edginess, disturbed sleeping pattern and complaints of feeling washed out, especially at weekends, when most people perk up.

What to look out for The following symptoms may be due either to diabetes or depression:

- exhaustion for no reason
- loss of appetite
- loss of libido, which means you don't feel like sex or notice anyone sexually attractive
- weight loss.

If these apply to you, have your diabetes checked, but be prepared to accept the possibility that they are expressions of your state of mind and can't be cured simply by means of better glucose control.

The following are additional symptoms that tell you that the thinking and feeling part of you needs help:

- you can't sleep properly and even when you do sleep heavily, you wake unrefreshed
- your concentration is poor – your mind wanders off when you are reading, listening or watching television
- your physical and mental energy levels are near zero, everything is an effort and nothing seems worth while
- you reduce your activities to a minimum
- your interest has evaporated, in, say, politics, music, friends and family and, finally, your appearance
- you feel so low that the idea of going to bed and never waking up may seem quite attractive
- you can't relax.

Penny was in just such a state. She was 34 and had been diabetic since the birth of her twins. She managed her part-time job as a receptionist, the demands of the children, now six, and running the home without much help from Bill, because of his job.

Then the depression came. Everyone in the family suffered, but Penny herself suffered most of all. In the end, she asked her doctor for something to help her sleep. She was dismayed when, instead of writing a prescription, she first of all checked Penny's blood sugar (which was satisfactory), then wanted to talk about what could be keeping her awake. Of course, Penny said everything was fine – the children were well, her marriage was happy, they had no desperate money worries.

There was one thing, however, her mother-in-law's proposed visit over Christmas. Bill was so looking forward to having his mother to stay that Penny could not say what she felt. The twins' routine would be completely disrupted. The older woman's views on childcare were diametrically opposed to Penny's. For one thing, she disapproved of Penny's job – 'a woman's place . . .' Dr Jones, herself a mother, instilled into Penny the confidence to explain her feelings to Bill and negotiate a shorter visit from his mother. Penny also had a course of stimulating antidepressants of the Prozac type.

Measures to combat depression Tranquillizers and sleeping tablets, especially the benzodiazepines, are essentially depressants and best avoided, except for a few nights to break a pattern of poor sleep. Instead of tablets, the best treatment is daily doses of outdoor air and exercise – no snoozing over the TV in the evening or daytime rests 'to make up' for a bad night – simple-to-cook and easy-to-digest evening meals and no cigarettes, alcohol or coffee late in the evening. Cigarettes and coffee are stimulants and while alcohol helps you to get off to sleep, its effect wears off in the small hours, leaving you feeling worse when you face the day. A warm bath and a hot, milky drink may help you settle down to sleep more naturally.

If you work outside the home, it is better to carry on if you possibly can. The social contact and useful occupation of your time are beneficial in depression.

PSYCHOLOGICAL HELP This can be in the form of expert psychotherapy or simple counselling during a difficult period and is readily available in American diabetic clinics. In Britain these facilities are patchy, but always available if you ask.

MEDICATION Antidepressants can speed your recovery and they are not habit-forming. The commonest type, the tricyclics, like Tryptizol, are not suitable for diabetics who are over 40, because their side-effects can cause eye or blood pressure problems. Less importantly, but still annoying, they tend to cause constipation and an increased liking for sweet foods. The newer classes of antidepressants have none of these disadvantages.

Anxiety

It is natural to feel some anxiety about your diabetes, but for most of us it only occurs when there is some new, special problem to focus on. Apart from the uncomfortable emotion, anxiety can show itself in a thumping heart, trembling, undue perspiration and nausea. All these symptoms could also be caused by hypoglycaemia (a shortage of glucose) if you are on insulin. Some people are in double jeopardy: they are frequently anxious about running into a hypo.

For this, and for any physical cause for anxiety, the first essential is information, while the second is support. The British Diabetic Association publishes a series of booklets on coping with specific problems (for their address, see the useful addresses section at the back of the book). These make a useful back-up to person-to-person discussions. Worrying about insoluble problems, like age itself, is a luxury it is best to learn to do without.

Eating disorders

Young women and teenage girls with IDDM are at above average risk of developing anorexia nervosa or bulimia – 7 per cent in each case, compared with 1 per cent among other girls. Males can be affected, but only rarely.

Eating disorders are a way of expressing conflict within the family, particularly between the girl and her mother in the younger ones or between a young woman and her boyfriend or husband.

The emphasis on carefully choosing food and self-control over diet that are necessary for dealing with diabetes can give eating exaggerated prominence in a young diabetic's mind. Experimenting with what she eats is not as dangerous as manipulating the insulin dosage as a slimming aid.

If you or your daughter have slipped into an overpowering obsession with food and weight, expert help is needed urgently. See a specialist at an eating disorders clinic.

Needle phobia

A phobia is a paralysing fear of something that you realize does not frighten other people. Examples are spiders, heights – and needles.

Needle phobia is obviously disastrous in IDDM as injections of insulin and blood tests are vitally necessary. If you have this phobia you cannot 'pull yourself together' without help, but psychological treatment will always effect a cure.

Obsessional neurosis

It is understandable – indeed your doctor recommends it – that you should be conscientious and precise about your diabetic self-care. This applies in both IDDM and NIDDM. For *meticulousness* to turn into *obsession* only requires a thoughtful personality and an upsurge of anxiety, from whatever cause.

An obsessional feels compelled to check and re-check all they do. This means that everything takes much longer, until, in the end, ordinary life is impossible.

This crippling neurosis will respond well to behavioural psychotherapy, when you will learn to stop carrying out the checking rituals.

Medication is sometimes helpful, if you are depressed as well as obsessional.

Alcohol and drugs

Diabetics are no more saintly than any other group of people, but at greater risk. Playing around with social drugs and drink rocks the physiological balance, which is the main aim of diabetic treatment.

Paddy's friends all like a drink. In fact, it was their chief leisure activity. Paddy's diabetes was a serious social nuisance, so he tried to ignore it or circumvent it by playing around with his insulin.

The result was a series of mini-disasters. He was in and out of hospital with hypos, ketoacidosis, infections and abdominal upsets so often that his boss decided 'regretfully, to let him go'.

At first, Paddy was defiant and drank all the more. Then the eye symptoms he experienced pulled him up short.

At present, he isn't drinking at all and he has stayed out of hospital for three months so far. He has had laser treatment for his eyes and is hopeful about getting a new job.

Some young people who dabble in drugs and drink are mistakenly labelled 'brittle diabetics'.

Brittle diabetes

This means having such an unstable metabolism that steady control of the diabetes is next to impossible. Life becomes a roller-coaster of good days and dips into illness.

There is a psychological element in brittle diabetes. The typical sufferer is a mildly overweight emotional young woman in her twenties, whose lifestyle is dominated by her illness. The danger lies in just accepting the situation without making the effort of a hard, consistent struggle necessary to win control of the situation. What is needed is frequent self-testing and care over diet and insulin dosage within the framework of a regular routine.

Children

When a child has diabetes, it is a family affair, and the youngster may prove to be a handful. Children express their feelings of anxiety, frustration or sadness in terms of what they do, so they may exhibit difficult behaviour, sulking on the one hand and devil-may-care naughtiness on the other.

For the parents, usually the mother especially, it means giving limitless time and patience, listening and explaining, plenty of love and understanding and unwavering firmness concerning those things that are important for the child's health.

The school must be warned against keeping a diabetic pupil in late, if it is likely to delay the child's meal or a routine insulin injection. Sport is an essential part of school life, which a diabetic child should not miss out on. It will help him or her to overcome any difficulties in mixing normally with classmates. Supplies of food may be needed to eat before or after a period of physical activity. Try this out at home first.

The greatest benefit parents can bestow on a child or teenager with diabetes is the restoration of self-esteem. The diagnosis will have made it plummet. Raising confidence calls for lavish doses of praise and any criticism should be expressed positively, as an alternative suggestion rather than a telling off. All young people experiment, so be prepared, not shocked or angry. This is especially relevant during those terrible teenage years, when authority is an Aunt Sally and mothers are barely tolerated, albeit affectionately. Expect to have alarm calls, times when you have to drop everything to deal with a hypo or cope with incipient ketoacidosis.

Checklist for parents

Think about the last week, then answer the following questions.

- How often did you praise your child for keeping to his or her diet, without cheating?
- How often did you nag your child about glucose tests or keeping his or her room tidy?
- How often did you congratulate your child for following a healthy self-care regime?
- How often did you praise your child for taking part in organized games?
- How often did you compliment your child on his or her appearance?
- How often did you ask for their opinion on any subject?
- How often did you admire something he or she had done?

Children are precious, but there would be no children without parents. Parents are important, too. The strain of a child's diabetes usually falls particularly heavily on the mother. It helps if you are calm and relations in the home harmonious.

Glenda had three children – Jane, Lucy and William. William was the youngest, the only boy and the only one with diabetes. It had started when he was seven. Glenda and Jack could not believe that it was happening to their family. They were riven with guilt, especially as a supply teacher had told Jane that diabetes was caused by an unhealthy diet.

When Glenda read about it (books on diabetes were her main reading matter these days), she realized that the way she fed the family *couldn't* be to blame for childhood diabetes. She reviewed all the illnesses experienced by grandparents, aunts and uncles. What would the future hold for their boy?

The worry kept Glenda awake. Although she was doing exactly what William's specialist advised, she felt helpless and incompetent. She imagined William dying an early death because of some mistake on her part. Her attitude towards him changed from jolly and unsentimental to anxiously solicitous. William didn't like it, and Jane and Lucy felt left out. Glenda lost her appetite and started losing weight. She was often in tears. Jack was bewildered, and buried himself in his work.

Glenda was one of the 23 per cent of mothers with a diabetic child who fall into a clinical depression. The danger is that it will drag on because no one realizes. In Glenda's case, it was her best friend who spoke to Jack, who spoke to their GP. Glenda recovered her perspective with treatment, which included plenty of opportunities to discuss her fears and feelings.

12

What to eat

As a diabetic, what should you eat? The answer is a normal, healthy diet, such as nutritionists all over the world advocate for normal, healthy people. The time has long passed when having diabetes meant eating special foods and never being able to share a meal with friends or even the family without standing out as 'different'. Of course, like anybody else, if you have high blood pressure, heart or artery problems or are unmistakably overweight, you must trim your diet accordingly.

The first step

Eating is part of everyday living and calls for a practical approach. First, you need to assess where you are now – your nutritional status. Check where your statistics come on the chart on page 118. You may also like to work out your body mass index. To do this, take your weight in kilograms and divide by the square of your height in metres. Acceptable index figures are 20.1 to 25 for a man and 18.7 to 23.8 for a woman. For a man a figure of 27 and for a woman a figure of 25 means that you are 20 per cent heavier than you should be.

There arc two basic types of diet:

- maintenance
- reducing – with a few modifications for special situations.

If you come into the 'just right' range on the chart or with your body mass index, you need the maintenance diet to keep you there. If you are underweight, as many of us are when we are first diagnosed as having IDDM, the shortfall is likely to correct itself once the treatment is well established, but you can add for instance an extra potato at supper or an extra slice of toast at breakfast until you get up to normal. There is no urgency.

If you are overweight, like 75 per cent of those who have just discovered that they have NIDDM, you need to work your way gradually on to the reducing diet. If you are in either of the two heaviest groups, you need to start this process at once, before the surplus fat has

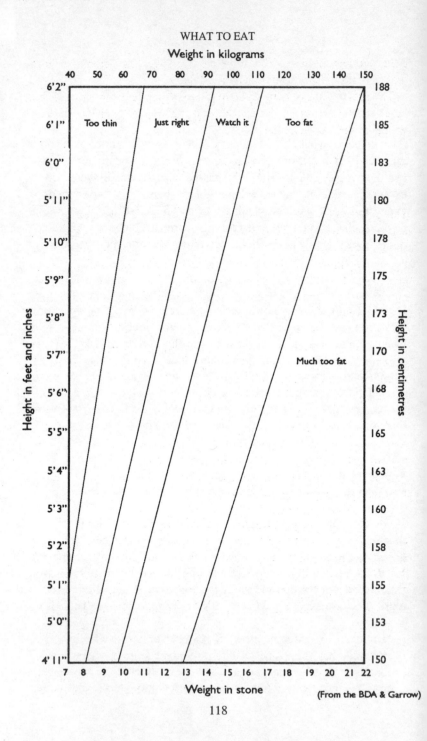

Weight in kilograms

Height in feet and inches

Height in centimetres

Too thin   Just right   Watch it   Too fat

Much too fat

Weight in stone

(From the BDA & Garrow)

118

done you lasting harm. The guidelines on page 121 will help you to work out how many calories you need daily.

The proportions of carbohydrate (50 to 60 per cent), protein (12 per cent) and fat (30 to 35 per cent) are the same whatever the diet and whatever the calorie value.

The basics of diet

Calories

The percentages of carbohydrate and so on just mentioned refer to calories *not* weight. Calories are properly called kilocalories and are shown as kcals on food labels. A single kcal is equivalent to 4.2 kilojoules of energy. The standard method of labelling food gives the kcal value for 100 g (4 oz) of the food and the proportions of each nutrient to be found in it. Here are some examples of the calorie values of common foods:

- apple, orange, pear, small banana or 10 grapes (100 g/4 oz) = 50 kcal
- cheddar cheese (100 g/4 oz) = 400 kcal (it has a high fat content)
- boiled or poached egg = 70 kcal
- fried egg = 130 kcal (high fat content)
- tablespoon of oil = 100 kcal
- slice of large loaf = 80 to 90 kcal
- boiled or baked plain potatoes (100 g/4 oz) = 80 kcal
- chips (100 g/4 oz) = 240 kcal (high fat content)
- fruit scone, without butter or margarine = 210 kcal
- small sponge pudding = 340 kcal
- meat: – small portion (50 g/2 oz) = 105 kcal
        – large portion (100 g/4 oz) = 210 kcal
- glass of wine = 75 kcal
- half pint of beer = 90 kcal

What some other diabetics eat

Below are examples of the two types of diet to give you an idea of how they differ.

An example of a Maintenance (normal) diet

Isobel was 32, a dealer in a firm of merchant bankers. She played badminton three times a week. She had had diabetes for six years and came into the 'just right' category for weight.

A typical day's meals for Isobel were as follows.

- Breakfast:
  - half a grapefruit (no sugar)
  - two slices of wholemeal toast with a scraping of low-calorie soft cheese
  - coffee with semiskimmed milk
  - muesli was her next favourite breakfast.
- Mid-morning:
  - coffee with milk, at work.
- For lunch:
  - an egg and tomato sandwich
  - a low-fat yogurt
  - banana
  - coffee.
- Mid-afternoon:
  - tea with milk
  - a biscuit or two.
- For an evening meal:
  - a lamb cutlet
  - potatoes, beans and carrots
  - fruit crumble
  - coffee.
- Late evening:
  - low-calorie chocolate drink.

At the weekends, when her boyfriend, Bob, was around, it would change a bit.

- For breakfast:
  - the same as usual.
- For lunch:
  - a quarter-pounder hamburger for Bob, a smaller one for Isobel, in a wholemeal bun if possible, with salad
  - fruit and ice-cream for him, yogurt for her
  - coffee.
- For an evening meal:

- meat and vegetable casserole, using 1 tablespoon sunflower oil and 1 tablespoon flour for the gravy
- jacket potatoes
- apple charlotte – cream with Bob's
- glass of wine.
- Between-meal drinks with semi-skimmed milk.

An example of a Reducing diet This is the health-saver diet, especially if you have NIDDM. Don't aim at peeling off the unwanted weight like an overcoat – a good rate of loss is 3 to 4 lbs (1.5 to 2 kg) per month. Most women need to work down towards a calorie intake of 1,000 to 1,100 kcals daily; for men it can be 1,100 to 1,300 kcals. Either way, you can't cope with cutting down all the way straight away.

SOME TIPS

- Don't be disheartened if you lose a lot to start with and then hardly any for a couple of weeks. This is because the early loss is mainly fluid and, although you are actually shedding fat after that, the water returns and evens up your weight on the scales.
- Make a record of all you eat and drink every day, then you will soon see what has gone wrong if you don't lose weight and what circumstances upset the plan.
- Never use food as a reward for successful dieting, but do give yourself other rewards for, say, every 2 kg (4 lbs) you lose.
- Make dietary changes step by step, not all at once.
- Remember that regular, moderate exercise speeds the slimming process, but, again, don't go from one extreme to the other.
- Never snack while in the kitchen or driving your car – extra calories tend to pile on unnoticed that way.
- Avoid like the plague any diets hyped in the media or small ads. They could make you ill, even if you hadn't got diabetes, and there is the further disadvantage that, largely, they only work temporarily.
- High-fibre foods are filling, but not fattening. Go for beans, vegetables, oats, wholemeal bread, pasta and so on, and fruit.
- Fats and concentrated sugary foods are the only real enemies.

Betty was exceedingly overweight – 50, fat, friendly and given to wearing bright colours – a delightful extrovert. She loved having people to the house and was generous in her entertaining. She smoked about 20 cigarettes a day and enjoyed a sherry in the evening before she got down to her ultimate pleasure – cooking. This involved a good deal of tasting.

Betty was inclined to deny that her diabetes mattered as she had more energy than most women her age, although her 114 kg (18 stone) made her puff going upstairs. To pacify her doctor, she said she would go on a diet. In her book 'diet' meant eating some fruit after her normal meals and trying not to have seconds.

Then crisis struck – just when she was extra busy preparing for Christmas. She thought it was indigestion as it came on after dinner, but the pain was excruciating. Betty got over her coronary – for that was what it was – but she remained at risk from the artery disease. Added to that, X-rays showed that she had mild emphysema.

She had to stop smoking straight away but her diet was more of a problem. Her regular sherry and having wine now and again were put on hold, long-term. Alcohol is not only full of calories, especially sweet sherry, but interferes with the metabolism in such a way that the fat stores are preserved. The major problem was what could Betty eat without spoiling her whole, expansive way of life?

Betty's interest in cooking was a plus here. She was able to work through the diabetic cookbooks from the BDA, including the slimming one, and found that the meals she produced were appreciated just as much by her guests as were the calorie-laden goodies she had provided before.

When she got into the swing of her diet, after a few weeks, a typical day went like this.

- For breakfast:
  - fruit juice, unsweetened
  - porridge with skimmed milk
  - Canderel sweetener to sprinkle
  - black coffee, if any
  - in summer she had brown toast with a sliced banana on top, no spread.
- Mid-morning:
  - an apple
  - coffee with skimmed milk
- For lunch:
  - a jacket potato with cottage cheese
  - salad, without dressing
  - a low-calorie soft drink

  – in summer she had an egg salad with a granary roll, and a drink.
- Mid-afternoon:
  – tea with skimmed milk
  – cracker or Ryvita, plain.
- For an evening meal:
  – a grilled chicken breast
  – ratatouille (made using 1 tablespoon of oil per 100 g/4 oz)
  – a hot wholewheat roll or some brown rice
  – a baked apple (with a sultana filling for guests)
  – a low-fat plain yogurt (cream or ice-cream for guests)
  – sparkling mineral water (white wine for guests)
  – at other times, spaghetti Bolognese, made using lean minced beef, or Quorn for vegetarians, vegetables, tomato purée and no fat, and wholemeal spaghetti; followed by fresh fruit jelly, with a topping for guests.
- Late evening:
  – tea with skimmed milk or a low-calorie chocolate drink.

A VARIATION If, like Saeed (see page 51) your blood pressure is high and you have some surplus weight as well, you need a low-fat, high-fibre reducing diet with low salt content, eating and enjoying as much as you like of the following:

- vegetables
  – anything green, all salad vegetables
  – tomatoes
  – carrots, swedes, turnips, parsnips
  – celery, celeriac
  – marrow, aubergine, artichoke
  – cauliflower
- fruit
  – grapefruit
  – gooseberries
  – rhubarb
  – cranberries

Note: put a mild limitation on all other fruits, fresh or cooked, without sugar.

- seasoning
  – pepper, mustard, vinegar, herbs, spices

- stock cubes, pickles, if they are not sweet.
- drinks
  - tea, coffee, Bovril
  - diet soft drinks, unsweetened fruit juice, sugar-free squashes.

Think carefully about all the extras in your diet.

- *Salt* Most of us take too much salt and it is definitely harmful if you have a tendency to high blood pressure. Don't sprinkle it on your food or add it to cooking and be moderate in your consumption of highly salted foods, such as bacon, cheese, processed meats, smoked fish, consommé, Marmite, Bovril, pickles and sauces.
- *Sweeteners* You ought to cut down on added sugar, but your tastebuds may not agree. Sweeteners such as sorbitol or fructose can cause stomach and bowel upsets when taken in excess and anyway they still add to your calorie count. Aspartame and saccharin contain no calories and do not have side-effects, but saccharin has a bitter after-taste, so aspartame is the most popular option.
- *Alcohol* It contains more calories than sugar, but offers no useful nourishment. If you are overweight, cut it out altogether if possible or be moderate even if you are not overweight. As with food it is more harmful to your metabolism to have a one-night binge than to drink the same amount over a longer period. Never take an alcoholic drink on an empty stomach as it is a quick route to hypoglycaemia.

'Diabetic' foods

Pharmacists, healthfood shops and ordinary supermarkets often display a range of foods labelled 'suitable for diabetics'. As you would expect, they tend to cost more than the ordinary equivalent. It would be worth the extra if there was a real advantage in using them. However, a *Which?* survey carried out in June 1994 showed that many of them contained just as much fat and contained just as many calories as other foods not labelled 'diabetic'.

For example, After Eights contained half the fat and only a few more calories than the special Holex After Dinner Mints at a third of the price of the Holex version. Boots' Diabetic Rich Fruit Cake included more fat and almost as many calories as Sainsbury's standard Rich Fruit Cake, while Sionon Diabetic Chocolate Cream Biscuits actually topped Budgens' ordinary bourbon creams for fat content and calorie value – at six times the cost of Budgens' biscuits.

It is not all bad, however. Sugar-reduced jams and marmalade are useful, so long as the sugar has not been replaced with sorbitol or fructose. Low-fat yogurts and sugar-free soft drinks are also worth buying.

Diabetics have been trend-setters regarding diet as we have been the first to settle for the healthiest combination of foods for all of humankind in this modern age, when stress is high and physical effort at a minimum. The others will follow.

Appendix
What do you know?

Read the following statements and put a *tick* by those you think are *correct* and a *cross* by those you think are *wrong*.

1 You can have diabetes without any symptoms.
2 Smoking is no more harmful just because you are diabetic.
3 It's a waste of time to go for a routine check if you feel perfectly well.
4 People with diabetes should not drive.
5 Hygiene and foot care are essential, even if you have no problems.
6 If you don't need insulin, it means you have a mild type of diabetes.
7 A crash diet is the best way to lose weight.
8 It is more harmful to have an occasional alcoholic binge than to have a drink every day.
9 Emotional stress affects your glucose level.
10 So long as they don't hurt, you need not worry about your feet.
11 People with diabetes all die young.
12 Diabetics can do most jobs, enjoy sport, marry and have children and lead a normal social life.
13 It is your fault if you develop diabetes.
14 Diabetes doesn't affect the brain.
15 If you are diabetic, you can never eat anything sweet again.
16 Fatty foods are more harmful to overweight people than carbohydrates.
17 Your children are at a high risk of diabetes.
18 You have special rights as a diabetic.

Turn to page 128 for the answers.

The Answers

1 Right. This is so to start with, but it helps to be alert.

2 Wrong. Smoking greatly increases the risk of heart and artery disease in diabetics.

3 Wrong. Most complications, especially those affecting the eyes, creep up silently.

4 Wrong. Most diabetics can drive when their illness is under control.

5 Right. Your skin and feet are vulnerable to injury and infection so you need to look after them.

6 Wrong. NIDDM is different to IDDM but it is just as dangerous.

7 Wrong. It upsets your metabolism and the weight does not stay off.

8 Right. It upsets your blood sugar.

9 Right. It increases your glucose level.

10 Wrong. If the nerves are damaged you may not feel if there is a further problem.

11 Wrong. Even without the expertise we have now, diabetics can live long healthy lives. H. G. Wells, for example, was diabetic and lived into his eighties. Many live this long or longer.

12 Right. It may take a little more planning, that's all.

13 Wrong. You can't choose or change your genes and constitution, so it is no one's fault.

14 Right. But, you may be temporarily confused during a hypoglycaemic episode.

15 Wrong. It is just a matter of exercising moderation.

16 Right. Fatty foods are more than twice as fattening as carbohydrates.

17 Wrong. The only exception is if *both* parents have NIDDM.

18 Right. A special Patients' Charter for diabetics in Europe laid down your rights in 1991.

Useful addresses

United Kingdom

British Diabetic Association
10 Queen Anne Street
London W1M 0BD
Tel: 0171–323 1531
Care line 0171–636 6112

Diabetes Foundation
177A Tennison Road
London SE25 5NF
Tel: 0181–656 5467

Ireland

Irish Diabetic Association
82–83 Lower Gardiner Street
Dublin 1
Tel: 353–1 363022

Australia

Diabetes Australia
QBE Building
33–35 Ainslie Avenue
Canberra City
ACT 2600

or

PO Box 944
Civic Square
Canberra City
ACT 2608
Tel: 61–62 475655

Canada

Canadian Diabetes Association
78 Bond Street

Toronto
Ontario M5B 2J8
Tel: 1–416 362 4440

United States of America

American Diabetes Association
National Service Centre
PO Box 25757
1660 Duke Street
Alexandria VA 22314
Tel: 1–703 549 1500

Index